The Art of Veterinary Practice Management

By Mark Opperman, CVPM

Veterinary Medicine Publishing Group
Lenexa, Kansas
A Medical Ecomomics Company

© 1999 Mark Opperman, CVPM

Published by Veterinary Medicine Publishing Group, 15333 W. 95th St., Lenexa, KS 66219; www.vetmedpub.com. All rights reserved. None of the content of this publication may be reproduced, stored in a retrieval system, or transmitted in any form or by any means (electronic, mechanical, photocopying, recording, or otherwise) without the prior written permission of the publisher.

Printed in the United States of America
Library of Congress Catalog Card Number 98-61301
ISBN 0-935078-74-6

10 9 8 7 6 5 4 3
First printing: February 1999

Acknowledgements

First and foremost I would like to acknowledge my wife, Marcie. She calls me her rock, but she is really mine. She has made my life whole and meaningful. Marcie is the reason why I have a "10" quality of professional and personal life. Marcie is also partially responsible for the second most important aspect of my life, my children: Chelsea, Seth, and Aaron. I did not know true joy and happiness until I became a father. The love in my children's eyes has been my strength in many a hotel far from home. My wife and children are indeed what's most important in my life and what life is all about.

I also must thank my assistants Susan Rudolph and Diane Elsbury. They worked countless hours and have as much blood, sweat, and tears in this book as I. They are also responsible for the success of VMC Inc. as much if not more than anyone else.

I owe who I am to my mother. My father passed away when I was 3. My mother was very strong and dedicated her life to—if not sacrificed it for—her children. Ethel Opperman taught me the importance of family, family values, and balance. My two sisters, Risa and Allene, and I grew up in a warm and loving environment. I love you, Mom.

There have been many people who have impacted my life and my career, more than I will ever be able to remember or mention. First and foremost I must acknowledge Dr. Terrance Claypoole. He is the reason I got involved in this profession and he was a great role model and father figure.

Mr. John Velardo, a past editor of *Veterinary Economics*, gave me my first opportunity to lecture and write. He had a great deal of faith in me and saw something in me I did not even see in myself. That tradition has been continued by other editors of Veterinary Medicine Publishing Group, and to them I also owe a great deal of gratitude: Ms. Becky Turner Chapman, Ms. Renée Anderson, Ms. Marnette Falley, and the head honcho, Dr. Ray Glick.

Drs. Ross Clark and Martin Becker taught me a great deal by "walking their talk" and setting a very high standard. Mr. Gary Glassman is my best friend in the world and has always been there for me personally and professionally. Dr. Charles Wayner and Mr.

Fritz Wood are great friends and companions that have also taught me a great deal in work and life.

If I have learned anything over the years it is that life is too short. We are only on this earth a short time, and we have little time to make a difference. I hope that this book will help to make a difference in the field of veterinary practice management by helping veterinarians and practice managers learn to practice smarter, not harder.

I hope this book will help to continue to elevate the field of veterinary medicine so that it continues to be revered and respected. It is a profession that I am proud to be a part of and one that I have devoted my life to. It is, in a word, AWESOME. My thanks to everyone who has helped make this book a success.

Mark Opperman, CVPM

Contents

Chapter 1

How Do Clients Perceive Your Value?

Patients can't go home and brag to their owners about the great care they received from you and your team members. Instead, clients determine your hospital's value based on what they experience during their first encounter with your practice.

It's important to note, however, that perception of value is rarely based on the quality of the medical care. A practice can leave clients with a negative impression but in fact provide excellent care. With no basis for assessing the practice's medical capabilities, clients form their impressions based on everything else, starting with the way you answer the phone. To bond clients to your practice never lose sight of the following:

1. Initial client contact. I've called veterinary hospitals before and heard someone say, "All Pet Clinic. Hold on, please," followed by a click and silence. What kind of message does that send? It sure doesn't tell them you're ready and willing to serve them. Your initial contact with clients, whether over the phone or in person, sets the tone of your relationships.

To get off to a good start, I recommend that receptionists answer the phone with, "Good morning. All Pet Clinic. This is Mary. How may I help you?" All four parts are equally important: the salutation, the name of your practice, the name of the person taking the call, and an offer to help. A fitting and complete ending for every call: "Thank you for calling All Pet Clinic. I'm glad we were able to serve you today."

When clients come through your front door, are they greeted immediately? Assign a receptionist the role of client greeter. This person will be responsible for knowing which clients are coming in which day and acknowledging them as soon as they walk in the door. In some practices, the greeter also sits down with new clients to help them complete the new-client form, then gives them a hospital tour to show the excellent care their pets will receive. Studies indicate that the client-bonding rate improves significantly in hospitals with a client greeter.

It's just as important to acknowledge the pet. When clients arrive, the receptionist simply looks at the appointment book or medical record and says, "It's nice to see you, Mr. Jones. I see that Casey is here for his comprehensive physical exam and vaccination visit. Please have a seat and Cheryl, our exam-room assistant, will be right with you."

Don't forget that in the client's mind, there may be no greater sin than to call the pet a "he" when in fact it's really a "she," or vice versa. Avoid that mistake by color-coding your medical records. I suggest blue forms for male patients and pink for females. Use color coding to show other information at a glance, too. For example, use yellow forms for avian or exotic patients.

2. Signage. Take a look at your hospital sign. Does it look well-maintained? What feelings does it evoke? I've seen some practice signs that look more appropriate for a daycare center while others give the impression that the hospital went out of business years ago. The sign plays a critical role in clients' perception of value, so it should reflect your practice's personality and professionalism. Chapter 4 features an in-depth discussion of this important marketing tool.

3. Building exterior. When you turn in to your parking lot, what do you see? Is the area well cared for—or is debris scattered about and piles of feces just waiting to be stepped on? Do you see attractive landscaping or clumps of weeds? Is the parking lot well-surfaced or full of potholes? Are parking lines visible or non-existent? Does the outside of your building say that you run a high-quality hospital?

4. Reception area. The term "waiting room" is not appropriate because no one in a veterinary hospital intends to make clients wait.

As you look around your reception area, assess the following:
- Is the client seating comfortable?
- Are the walls and floor clean?
- Can you smell unpleasant odors?
- Do you see peeling paint or torn wallpaper?
- Are any ceiling tiles cracked?
- Are informational posters and pictures professionally framed and hung on the walls?
- Are all display areas well-maintained and professional-looking?

The reception area brings up another question: How long do you typically keep clients waiting for their appointments? The most common reason clients leave one practice for another is a long wait. Studies show that you jeopardize your relationship with clients if you make them wait more than 15 minutes between the time of their scheduled appointment and the time they see the doctor. Of course, many factors play a role in client retention, including whether a long wait time occurs infrequently or often. Nevertheless, the 15-minute rule is a good guideline.

5. Receptionist's work area. Is the reception counter neat and professional-looking? A disorganized desk speaks volumes, so be sure to scrutinize the medical-record system, traffic flow around the reception counter, placement of phones and computer terminals, and the efficiency of work stations.

Do you know the one phrase spoken in veterinary hospitals worldwide? "I can't find the medical record!" Misplacing records is a common problem, but why tell the client about it? The pet owner's natural reaction will most certainly be, "If you misplaced my pet's medical record, what's going to happen when I leave my pet here? Will you misplace it, too?" Instead of admitting incompetence, just start a new record. When the original turns up, you can consolidate the two.

Now consider the role of your receptionist—in my opinion, the most important position in a veterinary hospital. To show you just how much influence a receptionist can wield, let me tell you about a personal experience several years ago. I had just moved to Indianapolis. Many of my clothes had gotten dirty and wrinkled during the move, so I took them to a nearby dry cleaners. When I picked up the laundry, I was less than impressed with the results. I returned a week later with another load of clothes, reasoning that because I didn't know any other cleaners in the area, I'd try my luck again.

When I walked in the door, the woman behind the counter astonished me by saying, "Good morning, Mr. Opperman." When I told her I was surprised she remembered my name, she said, "But of course I remember your name, and I also remember that you like your shirts done with light starch." The woman, who I learned was Doddie, was absolutely right. It impressed me so much that for the 10 years I lived in Indianapolis I took my clothes to that cleaners—and for 10 years they did less than an optimum job.

Why did I keep going there? Because of Doddie. She made everyone feel as if he or she were part of her family. It was always a joy to go to the cleaners and be greeted with such warmth. Doddie is my definition of a first-class receptionist.

6. Team professionalism. Your employees must be knowledgeable about the veterinary profession and the services your practice provides. They also must look professional, and that's why I'm a strong proponent of staff uniforms. You don't have to use uniforms that employees in fast-food restaurants wear. Your staff could wear, say, matching sweaters with navy blue or khaki pants.

Be creative and choose uniforms that reflect your practice's personality. One successful hospital's employees look professional wearing khaki slacks and a starched white shirt with the practice's logo embroidered on the pocket.

Whatever uniform you choose, it should include name tags for all staff members. It's also a good idea to include the name of your practice and hospital logo.

7. Exam rooms. Neat and odor-free exam rooms are a must.

These rooms should be cleaned after every patient visit. Use a hand-held vacuum cleaner for hair and dust and a good odor-control agent. Visiting clients may notice a lot of things you don't want them to see—a puddle of urine in the corner, cobwebs on the ceiling, or posters taped to the wall—so sit in the client's chair and observe your surroundings.

Keep in mind that clients desire comfortable seating in the exam room and a hook for coats and purses. A stack of current magazines or pet-health brochures may reduce wait-time frustrations as well.

I recommend that your staff not take clients to the exam room until the doctor or assistant is ready to see them. Clients waiting in exam rooms perceive the wait to be longer than it actually is, perhaps because they feel they're in "solitary confinement." On the other hand, clients with a fractious pet may be more comfortable waiting in the exam room. Be attentive and responsive to each client's needs.

8. Doctor appearance. Clients won't be impressed seeing their doctor wearing a lab coat stained with urine or blood, so freshen up between appointments. One study indicates that clients consider male doctors to be most professional when they wear a clean white jacket and dress shirt. Dress pants and ties depend on the work environment. Clients prefer female doctors to wear a white jacket with a blouse and slacks or a long white lab coat with a dress or skirt.

For a professional appearance, the common denominator is the white coat. I suggest a white jacket with the name of the doctor embroidered on it and perhaps the hospital logo. Studies show that the doctor's per-client transaction and client-retention rate are significantly higher for veterinarians who wear a white lab coat and professional clothes compared to those who wear colorful lab jackets or don't wear a coat at all.

Pay attention to your body language around clients as well. Do you enter the exam room with a smile and greet both the client and pet? Do you explain what you're doing during the examination? Do you tell the client what needs to be done at the follow-up visit?

Here's a 10-point exam-room checklist for doctors:

1. Introduce yourself. "Hello, I'm Dr. Smith."

2. Talk to and touch the pet. "Hello there, Casey. I think you're happy to see me!"

3. Do something. Conduct the exam or explain a procedure.

4. Say something. Explain what you're doing during the exam.

5. Show something. Point out the pet's tartar build-up or show ear mites under the microscope.

6. Give something. Give the client a handout on heartworm disease or FeLV. Don't just hand over the bill!

7. Listen. Then ask, "Do you have any questions or concerns?"

8. End on a positive note. Reinforce the client's decision to accept your professional recommendations.

9. Client exit. Escort the client through the visit. Team members can make a visit more pleasant by having the bill and medications ready to go. Time is even more precious after the visit because every minute the client has to wait will seem like three or four.

10. Finishing touches. Do receptionists itemize the bill and go over it with the client before giving out the total? Does every client receive an itemized receipt? Does a staff member offer to help clients out to their cars? Attention to these details go far.

Impress clients with a super outpatient visit

Now that you've critiqued your practice in these eight areas, let's look at a real-world example. What would a super, value-building client visit look like? I believe great visits depend on the use of an exam-room assistant. An effective assistant can strengthen your clients' perception of value and increase a veterinarian's productivity by as much as 75 percent. Just think of all the things a doctor does on a daily basis that could be done by a member of the support staff: run routine laboratory procedures, prepare prescriptions, clip up hot spots, or be the only person responsible for client education.

Here's what a typical outpatient office visit looks like in a hospital that uses its healthcare team effectively:

1. Linda, the receptionist, pulls the patient file before the next client arrives for his appointment. When Mr. Jones walks in the door with his dog, Casey, she greets them like longtime friends.

2. Linda notes in the record the reason for Casey's visit, offers Mr. Jones a cup of coffee or a soft drink, and asks him to have a seat. She tells him that Cheryl, Dr. Smith's exam-room assistant, will be with him shortly and directs him to some client education literature placed conveniently near the reception desk.

3. Linda places the file in a wall pocket outside the reception area and pages Cheryl to tell her that Mr. Jones is ready.

4. Cheryl picks up the record and reviews Casey's medical history, noting that he came in for a comprehensive physical exam and distemper/parvo vaccination. She also notes that it's been more than a year since they ran a fecal and that, according to the record, Casey hasn't been on heartworm prevention this past year.

5. Cheryl enters the reception area and greets Mr. Jones and Casey, then asks them to follow her to the exam room. On the way, Cheryl stops at the platform scale, weighs Casey, and notes his weight in the medical record.

6. When they get to the exam room, Cheryl reviews with Mr. Jones what they plan to do for Casey that day, informing him that the dog also needs to have a fecal exam and a heartworm check and be placed back on heartworm preventive. She communicates her care and concern without coming across as pushy. If Mr. Jones chooses not to take advantage of the preventive procedures, Cheryl will offer him a handout on the topic that he can read at home.

7. Before leaving the exam room, Cheryl offers Mr. Jones the opportunity to watch an educational video, then excuses herself.

8. Cheryl draws up the vaccinations and prepares anything else that might be necessary for the visit.

9. Cheryl tells Dr. Smith that Casey is ready and gives her a quick run-down of what she discussed with Mr. Jones, including any information he gave her. Cheryl has learned that if she overlooks that step, Dr. Smith will ask the same questions—leaving Mr. Jones to wonder why he even bothered to talk with Cheryl.

10. Dr. Smith enters and greets Mr. Jones and Casey. After assessing the situation, she begins the exam. Cheryl restrains Casey and assists as necessary, leaving Mr. Jones free to listen to the doctor.

11. After the exam and vaccinations are done, Cheryl puts Casey on the floor. Dr. Smith asks her to read the fecal and heartworm check. If the heartworm check is negative, Cheryl will prepare the heartworm medication.

12. Cheryl does the routine laboratory tests and prepares and labels the medication. She also enters all the information into the computer as a held invoice.

13. Meanwhile, Dr. Smith reviews an exam-room report card with Mr. Jones. It tells him that a comprehensive physical exam was performed on Casey and documents any health concerns detected during the visit.

14. Cheryl returns to the exam room to give Dr. Smith the test results and Casey's medication. The doctor reviews the results with Mr. Jones and hands him the medicine. While going over the exam-room report card, Dr. Smith learns that Casey has a feline friend at home that has fleas, so she asks Cheryl to review flea-control recommendations with Mr. Jones.

15. Dr. Smith tells Mr. Jones and Casey good-bye, then excuses herself to write up the medical record. She then checks the computer to make sure all the information has been entered.

16. When Cheryl completes her client education, she escorts Mr. Jones and Casey to the reception desk and lets Linda take over.

17. Linda itemizes the client statement before giving Mr. Jones the total. After he pays, she gives him an itemized receipt and offers to help carry things or simply makes sure that Mr. Jones and Casey get to their car safely.

This scenario may seem idealistic, but exam-room visits just like this one occur in hundreds of veterinary hospitals across the country every day. When doctors can spend high-quality time with clients and render professional services, they make 10 minutes with the client seem like 20, or 15 minutes seem like 30. Plus, the client has been left alone only a few minutes during the entire visit. As a result, the per-client transaction and the client-bonding rate increase significantly.

You have taken the first step toward creating your "10" practice.

Evaluate your practice with a "mystery shopper"

In order to know how clients truly perceive your practice, you need to be able to look at your practice objectively, from your clients' point of view. One way to do so is to use a mystery shopper.

The "mystery shopper" concept is simple and used often by many other businesses and professions. An employee visits a neighboring practice with either the employee's own pet or the hospital's pet, then

Mystery Shopper Report

Name of practice visited: _____

Date of visit: _____

Type of service requested: _____

Veterinarian seen: _____

Please check off services offered by this hospital:

   ❏ Exotic/Avian Medicine   ❏ Boarding   ❏ Grooming

   ❏ Prescription diets   ❏ Pet supplies   ❏ Pet foods

   ❏ Obedience training   ❏ Other

When you made your appointment, how were you handled on the telephone?

_____

_____

Distance of the practice from our hospital: ___ miles

Describe the outside of the practice. What was your impression of the sign, parking lot, landscaping, and other aspects of the external environment?

_____

_____

When you entered the practice, were you greeted by the receptionist?

      ❏ yes   ❏ no

Comments:

_____

_____

Describe the appearance inside of the practice:

Reception desk: _____

_____

Client reception area: _____

_____

Product displays: _____

_____

Informational displays: _____

_____

Exam room: _____

_____

What was the appearance of the doctors and staff?

Receptionists: _____

Technicians: _____

Veterinarians: _____

Practice manager: _____

What was the overall attitude of the staff?

What was the overall attitude of the doctor(s)?

Were you seen on time for your appointment? ❑ yes   ❑ no

Please describe the "bedside manner" of the doctor(s):

Were you informed of other needed services and preventive vaccinations for your pet?   ❑ yes   ❑ no

Did the practice:

Have a hospital brochure or folder?	❑ yes	❑ no
Use an exam-room report card?	❑ yes	❑ no
Use an exam-room assistant?	❑ yes	❑ no
Display recommended foods?	❑ yes	❑ no
Use a video for client education?	❑ yes	❑ no
Have a photo mural in the reception area?	❑ yes	❑ no
Itemize your statement?	❑ yes	❑ no

Competitive fee analysis

Procedure	Practice's fee	Our fee
Comprehensive physical exam	$ _____	$ _____
Annual distemper vaccination		
Canine/Feline (circle one)	$ _____	$ _____
Fecal analysis	$ _____	$ _____
Feline Leukemia test	$ _____	$ _____
FELV/FIP vaccination	$ _____	$ _____
Rabies vaccination	$ _____	$ _____
Heartworm medication	$ _____	$ _____
Flea-control medication	$ _____	$ _____

Comment on the practice's fees and the perceived quality of service:

What do you think are the best aspects of the practice you visited?

What do you think are the weakest aspects of the practice you visited?

On a scale of 1 to 10, with 10 being highest, how did their practice rate? ___
From your observation of the other practice, what can we do to improve our hospital? _____

reports back to the practice regarding their experience, using a practice visitation report to highlight important areas. This report guides the evaluation by reviewing the entire out-patient visit, from the initial phone call to final payment. (See Figure 1, pages 9-10.) The employee should present the results at the next staff meeting.

A mystery shopper program can open eyes, not only the practice owner's but the staff's as well. And often the experience is reinforcing, because the staff learns that the quality of your practice greatly surpasses that of the competitor. Mystery shoppers I've worked with have returned saying, "The doctor didn't even do a comprehensive physical exam!" or "When the receptionist told me the total amount due, she didn't ask if she could itemize the services. That hospital doesn't come close to ours!"

Many times employees return with good ideas to improve client service and enhance the practice's perception of value. One hospital I consulted with sent a technician to visit a local practice. She was impressed that the doctor completed an exam-room report card. She also reported that the doctor had thoroughly verbalized the physical exam and spent time with her reviewing the medical history and his suggested preventive procedures. Previously I had tried to stress this very point to this practice but they had resisted the idea. But after experiencing it from the client's perspective, the practice realized its value, and doctors and technicians were eager to begin using exam-room report cards themselves.

A mystery shopper also can produce other benefits. I know of a group of veterinarians from a community who collaborate with mystery shoppers. As a group, they decided to have employees visit each other's hospitals. The visitation report would be shared not only with the shopper's own team but also with the team of the visited hospital. Because participating hospitals never know when a mystery shopper might walk in, they were especially vigilant to ensure every client had a positive experience. The anticipation of the mystery shopper kept everyone on his or her toes and fostered a healthy atmosphere of competition that benefited all the hospitals.

To initiate your own mystery shopper program, first develop a practice visitation form. Second, discuss the concept at your next staff meeting, and ask for volunteers to be mystery shoppers. Next, the chosen mystery shopper should contact another practice in your community to make an appointment.

Keep in mind that although the mystery shopper can request almost any type of service, he or she will experience only the "public" side of the practice, just as your clients would. Therefore, if the shopper brings in a pet to be neutered, he or she will only experience the admission and discharge process and maybe a callback. However, the shopper will be much more involved with an annual comprehensive physical exam and vaccination visit and will gain greater insight. Naturally, the practice should pay all costs, including the mystery shopper's time. Consider the expense as an investment that will earn substantial returns.

Discharging patients

Paying careful attention to the discharge process is key to building clients' perception of your services' value. Your team must show clients that all surgical procedures deserve—and receive—your time and attention. One way to make a lasting impression: Set discharge appointments so doctors can talk about the procedures performed and review discharge order forms with clients. (See page 24.) If clients don't understand the value of your services, they won't hesitate to take their pets to low-cost spay and neuter clinics. And if you teach your clients that routine procedures are "routine," they'll treat them as such—and underestimate their value.

How does your hospital rate?

If you were to rate your practice's perception of value on a scale of 1 to 10, with 10 being the best, what would your score be? Your answer is critical—it will tell you how much you need to improve your clients' experience. Most veterinarians rate their practices a 6 or 7. Whatever your score, think about ways you can raise it. Remember, no practice can afford to rest on its laurels. In Chapter 2, we'll discuss how to enhance your practice's perception of value by adding client-pleasing amenities.

Chapter 2

Enhance Practice Value With Client-Pleasing Amenities

How can your practice stand out from the one down the street? If you ask today's top CEOs to share their secret for success, you'd be astonished at how simple the answer is. *Exceed customers' expectations.* Leaders in every industry make it their business to understand what their clients expect, then strive to exceed those expectations.

In part, your clients' expectations depend on their perception of your practice and the value of service and care it offers. For example, let's say you need a hotel room. If you check in at a Motel 6, you'll expect basic necessities: a clean room, bed, telephone, television—and not much else. Now, say you enter your room to find the bed turned down and a chocolate on your pillow. Does this exceed your expectations? Of course! However, if you check in to a Marriott instead, you *expect* that attention to detail. In fact, if you didn't get turn-down service, noticed slightly torn wallpaper, or had limited cable access on the television at a Marriott, you'd be disappointed. You might even decide never to return.

What does this mean for your practice? The little things really do count. Still, you don't have to pave your parking lot in gold to keep clients happy; small, personal touches usually impress them most. Some simple gestures that make a big splash: set up a client entertainment center, create a kiddie corner, offer new-client gifts, use exam-room report cards, and make medical recalls. Here's how:

1. Create a client entertainment center. Help clients pass the time by establishing a small client entertainment center in your reception area that includes a television, VCR, reading material, coffee, and a small refrigerator with soft drinks and juice boxes. You can show Oprah or CNN or perhaps offer children's videos.

Another touch clients appreciate: a courtesy telephone with a separate toll-restricted line. As you design your center, remember that the goal for this project isn't to educate clients but to help make their visits more enjoyable.

2. Make your practice child friendly. Think about your average client. Studies show that this person is a woman with 1.7 children. Now put yourself in her shoes as she arrives at your practice, children and pets in tow. Do you make her experience a pleasant one?

Consider this scenario: Several years ago I took my daughter to the pediatrician. I was truly impressed as we walked into the clean and colorful waiting room. The receptionist greeted us immediately and called my daughter by her name. Before I knew it my daughter was no longer by my side. She had found a Lego table in the waiting area. I too found myself drawn to the children's area. In no time I was playing one of the video games. It seemed just a minute before we were called to see the doctor. In reality it had been 15 minutes. This practice helped us pass time in an enjoyable way. I would gladly return.

You don't have to turn your waiting room into a daycare center to have clients say the same about your practice. A small table, chairs, and several toys keep children happily occupied. Some veterinary hospitals with limited space just fill a laundry basket with toys. The effect is the same.

Think you don't need child area? I once consulted with a practice owner in Des Moines, Iowa, who said they didn't need a kiddie corner because they didn't have many clients who visited with their children. Now I could be wrong, but I'm quite certain many pet owners living in Des Moines also have children. It's more likely these families visited other, more child-friendly practices. If you don't make children a part of their pets' veterinary experience, their parents will go somewhere that does.

Another benefit: A kiddie corner can lessen the stress on your healthcare team. How? We all know that if you don't give children something to fill their time, they'll find something on their own. A kiddie corner grabs kids' attention, freeing parents and team members to focus on the pet's health.

3. Introduce your practice with a new-client kit. Most practices offer new clients a new-puppy or new-kitten kit. Now consider extending your appreciation to first-time clients regardless of their pets' age with a new-client kit. The first time a new client enters your door, you get an excellent opportunity to bond with that person and pet. And offering a customized new-client kit makes a memorable welcome gesture.

Start by including basic health-care information, a hospital brochure or folder, and samples of recommended food and shampoo.

Then customize the kit with pertinent information on the pet's species or age. For example, new clients who bring in older pets should get information on geriatric care, and clients who bring in a bird or iguana should get information and care recommendations on their exotic animals.

To make this new-client kit really special, you might include a small gift, such as a leash with your practice name printed on it or a collar with a pet identification tag. A feline practice could give new clients a cat carrier with the practice name printed on it, or an Equine practitioner could offer a hoof pick or brush. Whatever you decide, your goal is to acknowledge new clients and offer them special service from the first moment they walk in your door. Personalized attention, information, and gifts can make a lasting impression.

4. Give medical recalls a high priority. Without question, one of the most critical ways you can exceed clients' expectations is to call them back after you discharge their pets. Not only will your attention impress them, but you'll get vital medical information. I believe every client whose pet was hospitalized should get a call from the attending doctor or a staff member a day or two after discharge. Follow up other medical cases with a call three, six, or 10 days later to check on the patient and ask how treatment is progressing. Even if you've scheduled a recheck, clients appreciate the call.

Recalls do more than exceed clients' expectations. They're also a

V-C-M INC

REPORT CARD

For: _____

FIRST NAME _____

LAST NAME _____

DATE ____ / ____ / ____

Vaccination Program

☐ Up to Date
☐ Vac. Due: CORONA/PARVO ____ Bordetella ____ LYME ____ DHLP-P ____ Rabies ____ FCVR/C ____ Leukemia ____ FIP ____
☐ Vac. Given: CORONA/PARVO ____ Bordetella ____ LYME ____ DHLP-P ____ Rabies ____ FCVR/C ____ Leukemia ____ FIP ____

1. Coat & Skin

☐ Appears normal ☐ Itchy ☐ Bacterial Infection
☐ Dull / Dry ☐ Shedding ☐ Fleas (M, Mo, S)
☐ Scabs ☐ Matted ☐ Hair Loss
☐ Hotspot ☐ Tumors ☐ Pigment

2. Eyes

☐ Appears normal
☐ Discharge: L___ R___   ☐ Infection: L___ R___
☐ Inflamed: L___ R___   ☐ Cataract: L___ R___
☐ Eyelid Deformities   ☐ Lenticular Sclerosis
☐ Other _____

3. Ears

☐ Appears normal   ☐ Tumor: L___ R___
☐ Inflamed   ☐ Excessive Hair
☐ Itchy   ☐ Yeast Infect: L___ R___
☐ Mites   ☐ Bacterial Infect: L___ R___

4. Nose & Throat

☐ Appears normal   ☐ Inflamed Tonsils
☐ Nasal Discharge   ☐ Enlarged Lymph Glands
☐ Inflamed Throat   ☐ Other _____

5. Mouth, Teeth, Gums

☐ Appears normal   ☐ Gingivitis (Inflamed Gum Tissue)
☐ Broken Teeth   ☐ Loose Teeth
☐ Tartar Buildup   ☐ Pyorreah (pus)
☐ Ulcers   ☐ Tumors

6. Legs & Paws

☐ Appears normal   ☐ Nails Too Long
☐ Lameness (LF, RF, LR, RR)   ☐ Joint Problems
☐ Damaged Ligaments   ☐ Foot/Hair Discoloration

7. Heart

☐ Appears normal   ☐ Fast
☐ Murmur   ☐ Other _____
☐ Slow

8. Abdomen

☐ Appears normal   ☐ Abnormal Mass
☐ Enlarged Organs   ☐ Tense/Painful
☐ Fluid   ☐ Other _____

9. Lungs

☐ Appears normal   ☐ Breathing Difficulty
☐ Abnormal sound   ☐ Rapid Respiration
☐ Coughing   ☐ Other _____
☐ Congestion

10. Gastrointestinal System

☐ Appears normal   ☐ Abnormal Feces
☐ Excessive Gas   ☐ Parasites
☐ Vomiting Problem   ☐ Other _____
☐ Anorexia (appetite)

11. Urogenital System

☐ Appears normal   ☐ Recommend neutering
☐ Abnormal urination   ☐ Mammary tumors
☐ Genital discharge   ☐ Anal sacs
☐ Abnormal testicles   ☐ Enlarged prostate

12. Weight _____ lbs.

☐ Normal range   ☐ Thin by _____ lbs.
☐ Heavy by _____ lbs.   ☐ Other _____

13. Diet

☐ Excellent   ☐ Vitamins needed
☐ Good   ☐ Improvement necessary

Dogs

Annual Heartworm Test
☐ Negative
☐ Positive
☐ Recommended

Heartworm Refill?
☐ Yes
☐ No

Cats

Leukemia / Aids Test
☐ Negative
☐ Positive
☐ Recommended

Cats / Dogs

Annual Intestinal Worm Test
☐ Yes
☐ No
☐ Recommended
Result _____

Flea Control Needed
☐ Pet
☐ House
☐ Yard

☐ Diagnosis / Description
(Numbers below correspond to numbers above)

☐ Lab results by mail / phone / consult

☐ Injection given

☐ Start medication at bedtime

☐ Give second dose medication in 2 weeks on ___ / ___

_____
_____
_____
_____
_____
_____

Recommendations

☐ Stay on heartworm pills year round

☐ Bathing recommended weekly / monthly / other

_____
_____
_____
_____
_____
_____
_____

DR. _____

Need _____ in _____ days

great marketing tool. Experts say people will share a positive experience with six others, and everyone knows word of mouth is the best advertising you can get.

To ensure that you and your staff follow up, I recommend you link recalls to a computerized service code. For example, if you type in a surgery code you'd get a reminder to call the client the day after the pet is discharged.

A few years ago, my firm, VMC Inc., and Arthur Andersen Consulting conducted a study of the veterinary profession. The study, funded by a grant from Hill's Pet Nutrition and titled "The Dynamics of a Successful Veterinary Practice," analyzed 52 highly successful veterinary hospitals in the United States. We also analyzed these practices' clients and employees. We discovered that clients responded very positively to medical recalls. Based on this finding, we recommend doctors handle surgical cases with a callback the evening of discharge. Clients feel most apprehensive the first night home with their pets. By the next day, the surgery is old news and the client is no longer as concerned.

Exceed clients' expectations and get true value out of recalls by making them on the evening of discharge. Keep in mind, however, that you should give the client about three hours to get home and settled before you call. If you can't, the next day will be fine.

5. Use exam-room report cards. Another way to heighten your clients' perception of value and exceed their expectations is to use an exam-room report card (see Figure 2, page 16). This form outlines the steps the veterinarian took during the physical exam and emphasizes that the pet received thorough medical attention. It reiterates problems noted during the exam, forces the doctor to verbalize the physical examination results, and, best of all, enhances client compliance. It also increases the practice's per-client transaction figure.

To get the most value from this tool, follow these steps: Complete the exam, administer vaccinations, and conduct any needed tests or treatments. Place the pet on the floor or into a pet carrier, and tell the client, "Mrs. Rudolph, let me review with you the comprehensive physical exam I just completed on Kyle."

Place the report card on the examination table and review your findings with the client as you fill out the form. Be sure to note all normal and abnormal findings, and write out your specific recommendations. When you're done, give the client a copy. You also can adapt the exam report card to fit different species. See pages 158 and 159 for examples of equine and avian report cards.

File the original in the patient's medical record. I recommend using two-part NCR paper to save time and improve the quality of medical records being maintained.

It's critical that the doctor fill out the report card in front of the client and discuss it with him or her. Working through this process normally takes about three minutes—time extremely well-spent when you consider how much hands-on interaction with the doctor increases the client's perception of the exam's medical value. Don't delegate this task to a technician or an exam-room assistant, and don't fill out the report card in the back hallway, then pass it to a receptionist to give to the client. The point here is that the client wants information from the doctor. If you pass the information through another team member, you've wasted everyone's time.

6. Improve client correspondence. Want to blow clients away? Send their pets a birthday card. You probably have most pets' birthdays noted in your computer records, so use it. If you don't ask clients for their pets' birth dates, start now.

Other well-designed forms of client correspondence also can help you exceed clients' expectations. For example, new-client welcome letters, "Thank You for the Referral" cards, and sympathy cards and letters all elicit client loyalty. One idea: Include a questionnaire with new-client letters to get feedback on how you can exceed their expectations.

7. Use a graduated referral reward system. One great way to cultivate new clients is to implement a graduated referral reward system. We all know that one of the primary sources of referral in any veterinary hospital is word-of-mouth advertising. This system helps accelerate the process.

An axiom of basic psychology says that if you positively reinforce an action, that action is more likely to occur again. Therefore, if we reward clients when they make referrals, it's more likely that they'll make more referrals. Out of this premise grew the graduated referral reward system. Each client who refers another to your practice receives a special gift acknowledging the referral and thanking them for thinking about your practice.

To set up this system, first develop a list of reinforcements to use. For example:

First referral:	$5 discount off the next office visit
Second referral:	A coffee mug printed with your practice's logo
Third referral:	Movie rental gift certificate
Fourth referral:	Complimentary weekend of pet boarding
Fifth referral:	10 percent off the next office visit
Sixth referral:	Flowers delivered to the client's home
Seventh referral:	$40 gift certificate from your pet retail area
Eighth referral:	Gift certificate for complimentary grooming
Ninth referral:	Dinner certificate at an elegant restaurant
Tenth referral:	"Preferred client" status, entitling the client to a 10 percent discount on medical and surgical services for one year.

Once you develop the system, the next step is to put it into place. Track referrals by adding a line to your new-client form that asks, "Whom may we thank for referring you?" Receptionists must be diligent about obtaining this information. When a new client says the referral came from an existing client, the receptionist should pull the medical record of that client's pet and note on the front cover the name of the person he or she referred, the pet's name, and the date.

This way you keep an ongoing, accessible record of the number of referrals each client makes. The doctor and receptionist can reinforce this process when clients visit by saying, "By the way, Mr. Smith, I see that you referred Mrs. Rudolph to our practice. She came in July 27 with Fluffy. Thank you very much for recommending us."

These ideas aren't earth-shattering, but they're effective. Consider this: Most veterinary hospitals provide about the same medical services—physical examinations, vaccinations, surgery, dentistry, and radiology. So, what makes your practice stand out? It's some little thing the client experiences. All it takes is a little time and a lot of personality to knock clients' socks off with service.

Chapter 3

Effective
Communication

Ever wonder why some clients stop coming to your practice? One study asked 3,000 consumers why they stopped shopping at particular department stores. Sixty-eight percent said they disliked the attitude or indifference of an employee. On its own this fact is significant, but it has even greater value when you team it with the results from a study conducted by Technical Assistants Research Program (TARP). TARP looked at consumer complaint behavior and found:

1. Ninety-six percent of unhappy people never contact the business that upset them.

2. For every complaint the average business receives, it has 26 unspoken complaints—six of which are serious.

3. Noncomplainers are less likely than complainers to do business again with the practice that upset them.

4. Between 54 percent and 70 percent of complainers will do business again if the complaint is resolved.

5. Ninety-five percent of people who complain will return if the complaint is resolved quickly.

6. The average person having a problem tells nine to 10 other people. Thirteen percent tell more than 20 people.

7. Complainers who have had problems satisfactorily resolved tell an average of five other people.

In other words, for every complaint you hear, about 260 potential clients will hear about your "bad" service from a dissatisfied client. How can you ward off these troubles? The most effective approach is to fine tune the communication skills of every member of your practice team.

Communication has three integral components: verbal, nonverbal, and written. In this chapter, I'll offer suggestions to improve your team's skills in each of these areas.

Verbal communication: Turning thoughts into sounds

It's a fact: The lower and deeper your tone of voice, the more authoritatively you present yourself. Many listeners perceive a high voice tone as irritating and often assume the speaker is insecure. Think back to times when you've heard an upset person's voice get louder and higher pitched. What impression did that make? With a little effort, you can maintain a low, deep tone of voice and appear in control, even during the most heated disputes.

Another important aspect of verbal communication is timing—that short pause you use to accentuate your point. Professional speakers know the best way to get a noisy crowd's attention is to stand at the podium without saying a word. It's the same in your practice. Clients and employees expect you to speak. When you stop, they notice.

Make this work to your benefit in the exam room. You might say, "Mrs. Smith, let me review the discharge instructions with you. I recommend (pause) that you feed Casey small quantities of food and water this evening." The pause accentuates your recommendation.

Atmosphere also can affect your success. Experts estimate that inappropriate atmosphere causes 60 percent of communication failures. Employees feel a greater sense of accomplishment and pride when acknowledged in front of their co-workers. At the same time, it's best to discuss problems in private. If you are having constant communication problems, you may want to assess when and where you handle important conversations.

The way you talk makes a difference, too. Do speech impediments, accents, or language problems affect your clarity? If so, find ways to improve the problem, either with communication courses or speech therapists. Likewise, succinctness is critical. Consider this: A client

calls the practice to inquire about heartworm prevention. Do receptionists offer concise information, or do they chatter for several minutes to express a simple thought. Many practices make certain every
team member gives concise information to callers by using scripts for
routine calls. A number of receptionist training manuals make excellent sources for these scripts.

Take time to observe your staff's verbal communication. Ask a
friend to make an anonymous call inquiring about a preventative procedure to see how your staff performs. Clear, succinct communication means that clients go away with the answers they need—and
with the impression that your practice team is both knowledgeable
and professional.

Nonverbal communication: Actions speak volumes

Nonverbal communication, or body language, can account for up to
60 percent of your communication. In fact, when verbal and nonverbal communication send conflicting messages, people believe the
body language. Consider a veterinarian standing in a corner of the
exam room, arms folded and making no eye contact, who says, "Your
pet's health is my highest priority." The words say "concern" but the
body language says "I could care less."

Without realizing it, you probably send negative nonverbal signals
throughout the day: a wrinkled forehead, a pursed mouth, repeated
swallowing, excessively clearing your throat, or insincere smiles. Perhaps the most tell-tale nonverbal cues revolve around eye contact, or
lack of it. How often do you stare at clients, blink rapidly, shift your
head or eyes, or squint? Other negative gestures include covering
your mouth while speaking, scratching your head, rubbing the back
of your neck, preening, tinkering with jewelry or clothing, constantly
shifting your weight, pacing, freezing, crossing arms, and cocking
your head. You may even unconsciously take a hostile stance or look
down on someone.

Everyone does some of these things some of the time, but when
done to excess they become a problem. It's amazing how detrimental
negative nonverbal communication can be to your interpersonal relationships. Monitor your nonverbal communication and teach your
staff to do the same. Many practices find it helpful to team up

employees for a day to observe each other's verbal and nonverbal communication. At the day's end, the two can provide each other with constructive feedback and suggestions for improvement.

Written communication: Put it down on paper

Your practice's written communication is what clients generally carry away from the hospital, and these materials can make a big impact on the image of your practice. Do your client education and marketing materials show the world that you're a professional, high-quality healthcare provider? Are client education materials typeset and printed professionally—or are they repeatedly photocopied, leaving streaked text that clients can hardly read? Keep in mind, the way you present information can affect people's perception of the importance of the information dramatically.

It's also important to make sure you give clients the information they need, when they need it. For example, let's return to giving the client discharge instructions. Clients often need lots of information on caring for their pets after a hospital stay. Concise written communication can reinforce your recommendations—and head off calls from clients who can't remember all the instructions. If you don't already use a Discharge Order Form in your practice, consider designing one. This form should cover such pertinent information as proper restraint, food and water, diet, elimination, exercise and activity, medications, sutures, appointments, monitoring, and any special instructions. Check-off forms are the most user-friendly, and can include ample space to write in specific instructions for clients. (See Figure 3, page 24.)

Another excellent idea to streamline written communication: Develop and use a standardized estimate book. How many times in one week does your practice write estimates for an abscess? Don't reinvent the wheel each time! I recommend you create an estimate for all procedures. An estimate book saves your team time, and ensures that every doctor in the practice gives every client the same cost estimate for procedures, every time.

I suggest the practice manager and veterinarians design the estimate book. Start with an explanation of the procedure. This tells clients that the pet is more important than money (See Figure 4,

Care of Your Pet Following Surgery or Hospitalization

Pet's Name _____   Procedure _____   Discharge Date _____

PROPER RESTRAINT: Please protect your pet when leaving the hospital by using either a leash or a carrier. Excessive activity may result in your pet getting loose or result in injury if your pet is recovering from surgery. Do not allow your pet to become overly active and excited when you pick him/her up from the hospital.

FOOD AND WATER: With the excitement of returning home after surgery, your pet may be inclined to drink and eat excessively, which may likely result in vomiting. To avoid this, we recommend restricting access to water for an hour or so until your pet has quieted down. Then, allow only small amounts for the first 8 hours. Normal feeding may resume the next day.

DIET: If a special diet has been prescribed, please follow the instructions carefully:
☐ Feed your pet his/her regular diet.
☐ Feed multiple smaller meals _____ times per day.
☐ Special diet: _____

ELIMINATION: Many patients may not have a bowel movement for 24 to 36 hours after surgery. This is normal.

EXERCISE AND ACTIVITY: Patients recovering from surgery or illness should have limited exercise. Avoid access to stairs or situations that may lead to injury. Due to the affects of anesthesia, he/she may be groggy for 12 hours.
☐ Your pet may resume normal exercise and activity in _____ days.
☐ Your pet should be confined to indoors and taken outside on a leash only for eliminations for _____ days.
☐ Your pet should be under strict confinement to a cage or small room for _____ days. Carry outside for eliminations. No running, jumping or access to stairs is permitted.

MEDICATIONS: If dispensed, it is important to follow directions carefully.
☐ None dispensed.
☐ Dispensed, directions attached.

_____
_____
_____
_____

SUTURES: Discourage your pet from licking or chewing at the sutures. Please check the incision daily for any swelling, redness or discharge. If sutures appear irritated or infected, notify us immediately.
☐ Sutures will be removed by appointment _____ days from the date of surgery.
☐ Sutures are absorbable and don't need to be removed.

APPOINTMENTS: Please make an appointment for the following:
☐ Suture removal in _____ days.
☐ Drain removal in _____ days.
☐ Bandage/cast change/check in _____ days.
☐ Re-check in _____ days.

MONITOR: A decrease in activity or appetite for one or two days may be observed. However, if your pet exhibits any of the following symptoms, please notify the hospital:
(1) Loss of appetite for over 2 days (2) Refusal to drink water over 1 day (3) Weakness
(4) Depression (5) Vomiting (6) Diarrhea

SPECIAL INSTRUCTIONS:

_____
_____
_____

Abscess

An abscess is a pocket of infection that contains pus. It often results from a cat bite where the skin is broken and hair and bacteria are trapped under the skin. The wound then seals and the abscess develops. This is usually quite painful and your pet could be less active and have a fever during this time. Surgical treatment is sometimes necessary to drain the abscess, then your pet will be placed on antibiotics. With severe infection, your pet will possibly need to be hospitalized following surgery.

ESTIMATE OF COSTS FOR DRAINING ABSCESS

Examination	$ 32.00		
Anesthesia	69.00		
Draining and Flushing the Abscess	49.00		
Antibiotic Injection	21.00		
Hospitalization / Recovery	27.00	-	39.00
Antibiotic Medication Going Home	18.00	-	21.00
TOTAL:	$216.00	-	$231.00

If your pet needs to be hospitalized following surgery:

Hospitalization	$ 27.00		
Daily Doctor Professional Care	20.00		
Antibiotic Injection	18.00		
TOTAL:	$281.00	-	$296.00

above.) Next, outline a cost range for each element of the procedure, and describe any necessary costs should the patient be hospitalized. I don't recommend estimates that show a set fee; you need built-in flexibility to cover unexpected problems. Store the book in your computer and print out the appropriate page when needed, or keep a printed estimate book in each exam room.

A Surgical Consent Form is a third example of effective written communication. (See Figure 5, page 27.) This form combines a surgical consent with a laboratory test waiver. With this approach, you can promote pre-anesthetic laboratory workups but give clients the option of refusal if a patient is less than 6 years old. Most practices require patients older than 6 to have workups before they perform surgery.

The varying degrees of communication

To be an effective communicator, you need more than verbal, nonverbal, and written skills. You also must recognize that people communicate at different levels. Good communicators can assess others' reactions within the first 30 seconds by interpreting their body language. If you don't get an appropriate response, change your approach. Maybe your language is too complicated, or maybe the client is distracted or feeling upset and can't concentrate. Remember, it's your responsibility to ensure that others understand what you're trying to say.

Role playing is a great way to improve your team's communication skills. Present your staff with various situations and assign each a specific role. Besides helping resolve practice communication problems, playing the roles of clients and other team members can give participants more insight into other people's perspectives. The only rule: Players must reach a conclusion.

Staff meetings are a great time to try role playing, especially when you implement policy changes. At your next meeting, have your team enact this scene between a receptionist and client:

An angry client calls in, upset that your practice included a service charge on his account balance. He says that if you plan to charge this, you might as well mail him his pet's records because he's switching to another practice. The receptionist must resolve the situation. While two team members role play this scenario, ask remaining staff to observe the players' verbal and nonverbal communication and offer suggestions for improvement.

What do clients really want?

You know the ramifications of ineffective communication. The solution is knowing what people really want. People want others to appreciate them, listen to them, help them, use their name, be creative, and be honest.

Everyone wants to hear that they are important and appreciated. Tell employees exactly how you feel about them. Say "I appreciate...," "Thank you for...," or "It helps me when you...." Show clients your appreciation by always being polite, never judging them, and by all means, never challenging them. As you talk, remember that body language says more than words. Stand up to greet each client and, when appropriate, offer your hand.

People also want others to understand them. When a client voices concerns, don't just say, "I understand," but paraphrase the problem. For example, saying, "I understand you're upset because your bill is

Surgical Consent Form

Date _____ Pet's Name _____
Owner _____ Species _____
Address _____ Breed _____
                            Sex _____
Today's Phone Number _____

As the owner or agent of the owner of the above animal, I hereby give my consent to *[Hospital or Veterinarian Name]* to perform the following procedures:
1. _____
2. _____
3. _____

I understand that during the performance of this procedure, unforeseen conditions may be revealed that necessitate an extension or variance in the procedure(s) set forth above. I expect [Hospital or Veterinarian name] to use reasonable care and judgement in performing the procedure(s). The nature of the procedure and risks involved have been explained to me and I realize results cannot be guaranteed. I am also aware that unforeseen events resulting from the procedure(s) will not relieve me from any obligation to all reasonable costs incurred regarding the animal.

Signature of Owner/Agent

ALL ANIMALS ADMITTED MUST BE CURRENT ON THEIR VACCINATIONS AND MUST BE FREE OF EXTERNAL PARASITES. ANY ANIMAL FOUND TO HAVE FLEAS OR TICKS WILL BE TREATED AT THE OWNER'S EXPENSE.

Laboratory Tests Waiver

If your pet is to be anesthetized, rest assured that advances in anesthesia and surgery have made routine procedures relatively safe with a low rate of complications. Nevertheless, occasional problems can arise due to pre-existing conditions not evident during routine pre-anesthetic examinations. To avoid these problems, we recommend that all of these cases be screened prior to anesthesia by means of the following laboratory tests. These tests will be performed (and you will be billed for them) unless you refuse them by initialing and signing below.

Initial for Refusal:
___ A. White Blood Cell Count, Packed Cell Volume,
        Blood Clotting Time, Function Screen, Liver Evaluation $42.00
___ B. Leukemia Test (cats, if not tested within last year or vaccinated) $29.00
___ C. Heartworm Test (dogs, if not currently on preventive) $28.00

Signature of Owner/Agent _____

Receptionist _____

more than you expected" will convey empathy. Use the same words as the client and, when appropriate, sympathize with personal remarks: "I was at my doctor's office last week and she made me wait. It really upset me. I understand how you feel."

Ask questions to get more information, and react positively with gestures, facial expressions, and voice tone. Respond clearly with simple answers and avoid jargon. Remain objective. Probably the most important thing is to remember that clients are usually not angry at you, they are angry at the situation.

It only takes a minute longer to really help clients. Never refer to company policy—you're merely hiding behind the words and not resolving the situation. Whenever possible, go the extra mile and volunteer information before a client or employee can ask for it. There is a saying: The true test of intelligence is knowing how dumb you are. When you don't have the answer, say, "I don't know, but I will try to find out for you."

During all interactions, keep in mind that people enjoy hearing their name and respond favorably to those who use it. Use this to your advantage by saying the client's and pet's names often, but be sincere. Never fake a sweet voice and always be pleasant.

Last but most important: People want others to listen. Effective listening skills are an admirable trait. Experts say we spend 30 percent of our time speaking but 45 percent listening. Unfortunately most people listen at a 25 percent efficiency level. In other words, what you do the most, you likely do the worst.

Listening skills are critical for effective communication to occur. To become a good listener, you must prepare yourself physically and mentally. First, identify the purpose of the communication. Is it persuasive, informative, sharing, or social? Second, you must actively listen. Focus your eyes on the person, telephone, or even computer screen. Be mentally alert and overcome distractions. Finally, remain nonjudgmental and objective. React to the idea, not the person. Don't become irritated at what a client says or the way he or she says it. Good listeners don't jump to conclusions. They avoid making assumptions and don't complete sentences for others. Instead, they listen to what is being said, then respond to it.

As you work on your active listening skills, turn off your own worries and use such listening responses as "Yes, I see" and "I understand." Limit your own talking and clarify what has been said by rephrasing the conversation. Active listeners ask open-ended questions: who, what, why, where, and when. Listen to comprehend and interrupt only to ask questions. Think about how you'd feel if you were a client or employee. This approach can help you focus on the other's point of view. I recommend you take notes and ask lots of questions. It's vital that you don't do other tasks while talking to a client or employee. Give your full attention to the person.

I can't stress it enough: Effective communication is key to your practice's success. It's critical that you assess your team members' communication skills and help them improve upon those skills whenever and wherever possible.

Chapter 4

Educate Clients
With Marketing

Before you shudder at the thought of marketing your practice, realize that I don't mean blatant self-promotion. Marketing is a way to inform people about your products and services. A friend of mine defines marketing as putting your products and services at risk of selling them. In fact, I believe you are negligent if you refuse to market. Clients unaware of the many products and services available have limited choices, so you must advocate excellent pet health care.

Consider this fact: A study done before once-a-month flea control products were available found that consumers spent $240 million on flea-and-tick collars alone. How much of that was spent at veterinary practices? A mere 7.6 percent.

Anyone involved in this profession knows that collars purchased in a veterinary practice are more effective. So why did 92 out of 100 people waste money on an inferior product? Because an average person didn't know the difference. It wasn't until the veterinary profession used informational marketing to educate consumers that people knew their veterinary team could really help in the fight against fleas.

Unfortunately, not every product or service gets the benefit of aggressive, nationwide educational campaigns. That's why it's critical that *you* educate clients about preventive care. Marketing your products and services helps you do this.

There are two types of marketing: external and internal. External tools include your practice sign, hospital brochures and folders, target marketing campaigns, stationery, newsletters, and reminder systems. Internal marketing refers to new-client kits, client-education handouts and videos, special discount offers, and photo murals. In this chapter, we'll look at several tools you can use.

External strategies

Draw them in with an eye-catching sign
Your practice's sign can be an excellent external marketing tool, provided it does the following:
1. Identifies your practice
2. Creates an image
3. Improves your visibility
4. Provides information
5. Enhances the appearance of your practice

When selecting a design to represent your practice, remember that color has the biggest impact. Think about Burger King, McDonald's, Hardees, Wendy's, and Shell Oil Company. All use eye-catching red and yellow. Personally, I'm not crazy about yellow, but I do feel red is a powerful choice. Use red to accentuate the most important words on your sign. What is more striking than the words "Animal Hospital" in red on a white background?

A sign also should provide information about your services. Do you offer boarding and grooming? What are your business hours? Do you care for livestock or companion animals? Passersby don't care about the owner's name or even a phone number. Instead, they want to see what you can offer them.

Many practices use changeable letter boards in their signs. These can be effective, but I recommend you change the wording every week. The flexibility lets you provide more information to potential clients and keeps your sign fresh—well-worth the extra maintenance.

Let a professionally produced brochure do the talking
Hospital brochures are an impressive way to give clients the information they need about your hospital. For example, you can include a

philosophy statement about your practice and list the services you provide, such as physical examinations, vaccinations, dental work, emergency service, and so on. Be sure to include such ancillary services as boarding and grooming.

For big impact, include photographs in your brochure. For example, show a technician caring for a patient or a doctor performing a dental procedure. Your brochure should also inform clients about diagnostic services you offer, such as comprehensive radiograph services, full medical laboratory, allergy testing, and surgical procedures. A surgical-suite photo shows clients the technology behind your services better than any explanation.

Explain your policy regarding elective procedures, withholding food and water before hospitalization, prescription refills, hospitalization, and visitation. Many brochures also contain preventive health-care schedules for puppies, kittens, and adult animals as well as the practice's euthanasia policy. Finally, include hospital hours, doctors' hours, what to do in case of emergency, and your payment policy.

As a bonus, many practices incorporate a health record in their brochures. Your staff can note immunizations, fecal examinations, heartworm preventative, and even weight and growth on a chart. This approach makes the brochure a constantly used tool instead of a one-time only reference. Encourage clients to bring in the record regularly so your staff can update it.

Why invest in this expensive tool? Studies say that one client will show your brochure to five other people—be sure you're giving your clients the tools to publicize your practice.

Attract potential clients with a hospital folder
Want an easy way to convert telephone shoppers into clients? Send them a hospital folder. Before you brush off this idea, put yourself in the caller's shoes. When calling various businesses, you may have no idea of what makes one company better than another. But if one company sends you information that clearly demonstrates its commitment to quality, you'd be impressed. A nonscientific study done with several VMC clients found that during a one-year period, practices who sent out hospital brochures or folders converted a whopping *72 percent* of phone shoppers. Not bad, wouldn't you say?

The problem with brochures is that you can't update the information easily. For example, when you add a veterinarian or service, you have to reprint the entire brochure. That's where a hospital folder comes in handy. The cover lists the practice's name, logo, address, and phone numbers—information that's unlikely to change any time soon. Use the two inside pockets to hold staff information sheets and handouts about your services. Of course, professionally designed and printed sheets tell clients yours is a practice of high standards and quality, and well worth your fees.

The folder's flexibility lets you change information regularly. Even better, clients can use it to store their pet's medical information—an easily identified reference that busy people appreciate.

Once you've got the folder compiled, it's simple to get your marketing effort started. When people call to ask about vaccinations and elective procedures, train your receptionist to ask them if she can send information about the practice and its services. If they agree, send a hospital brochure and handouts about the services the person asked about that same day. Then sit back and wait for the calls.

You can also use hospital folders as client information packets to customize your education and marketing efforts. Tailor the folder to meet each client's specific needs, and consider including a little gift such as a wall magnet or pet bandanna to help bond your client to the practice.

Target marketing: Get information to those who need it
Target marketing lets you identify a client group with specific needs and then offer them a product or service they may be particularly interested in. Geriatric or dental services are excellent focuses for target marketing.

For target marketing to be effective, you must:

1. Identify a target group of patients.
2. Offer these clients a package of services that fits their needs.
3. Educate them about the service.
4. Provide them with an incentive to take advantage of the service.

Say you want to market dentistry during National Pet Dental Health Month. First identify all dogs and cats older than 4 years that have visited your practice in the past year but didn't have a dental

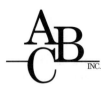

March 1, 1999

Mrs. Jane Doe
100 America Street
New York, NY 14025

Dear Mrs. Doe:

The field of veterinary medicine has changed over the years, and today your pet's life expectancy is greatly enhanced. Along with a longer life, your pet may experience more age-related diseases.

Because your pet is now considered a "senior citizen," we recommend a thorough physical examination. Just like in humans, early detection and treatment of diseases can help your pet live a longer life—and help us to maintain the quality of your pet's life.

We recommend a geriatric wellness exam, which includes a:

1. Comprehensive Physical Examination
2. Complete Blood Count
3. Chemistry Analysis
4. Urinalysis
5. Fecal Exam
6. Heartworm Test

The normal cost of this service is $140. As an incentive to encourage you to use this early detection system, we will provide this service for only $105, but only until May 1, 1999.

After the testing is complete or at the time of the examination, we will schedule a consultation either over the phone or in our office, to report the results of the examination to you and make our recommendations for follow-up care if needed.

Please call the ABC Veterinary Hospital for more information about your pet's geriatric work-up. Your pet's health is our primary concern.

Sincerely,

The Doctors and Staff of the
ABC Veterinary Hospital

prophy performed. Next, create an targeted letter you can mail to their owners. It should explain the importance of preventive dental care and note that February is National Pet Dental Health Month. As an incentive, you can offer a complimentary dental exam and 15 percent discount off a prophylactic treatment.

To round out your campaign, hang a poster about Pet Dental Health Month in your reception area. Another great idea: Create photo murals showing patients with severe periodontal disease before and after dental treatment, and hang them in your exam rooms.

Geriatric wellness also is an excellent focus for a target marketing campaign. In this case, you might identify all dogs and cats over 6 years old that visited your practice in the past year but haven't had a geriatric wellness exam. Design and mail a targeted letter to these clients. (See Figure 6, page 34.) As with the dental target marketing, consider posting photo murals and posters in the exam rooms.

Target marketing doesn't just build profit centers. More important, it helps you educate clients about vital veterinary services. Consider target marketing for nutritional counseling, feline leukemia, heartworm, and flea control. Some practices even promote a "vaccination amnesty" month for patients that are overdue for vaccinations.

Many practices initiate target marketing during slow months to spread client activity throughout the year. This approach means the practice is more profitable and can maintain a high-quality staff year-round—a factor that's essential to long-term financial success.

Other external marketing tools
Everything that comes out of your practice represents you and the medical quality you provide. Make sure the following business essentials reflect your high standards.

Practice newsletter
Newsletters alone can help bond clients to the practice but may not generate direct income. But this changes if you use them to enhance other marketing campaigns. The newsletter lets you put a bug in clients' ears about a certain preventive procedure. While they're considering the option, you hit them with a great incentive to try it out.

Here's how it works. Say you want to market dental services. Discuss preventative dental care in your newsletter, then follow up two weeks later with a postcard campaign that highlights Pet Dental Month and offers a promotional product or service.

I recommend large animal practices use newsletters on a semi-annual or quarterly basis. You can promote services and keep large animal clients informed about your practice. Again, however, you need to fully use other external marketing tools—reminder systems and hospital brochures and folders—before spending valuable time and resources on a newsletter.

Business cards and stationery

I can't stress it enough: Image is vital to your success. What represents you as a doctor and business owner more than your business card? If designed correctly, this marketing tool can provide clients with excellent information about the quality of your practice and services. I recommend fold-over cards. With this tool, you have twice the space to provide beneficial information. Make sure to include your logo on the front as well as your name, title, practice name, address, and phone numbers. The inside can list such information as special services, emergency instructions, and a brief description of your dedicated team.

Many practices offer magnetic business cards to new clients or make them available at the reception desk for clients to take. Clients love it and display it proudly on refrigerators or near telephones.

Pet bandannas

People love pet accessories. What could be better for you than clients who show off pets that are sporting a bandanna with your practice logo, name, and phone number? Many practices offer bandannas to reward clients who bring in their pets for their yearly comprehensive physical exam and vaccination. Yeah, it's anthropomorphic, but I swear I've seen animals leave with heads just a little bit higher and tails wagging a little bit faster. And nothing endears clients as much as their pet getting a little extra attention from you.

Community outreach programs

External marketing extends far beyond hospital brochures, reminder systems, and business cards. The best way to educate your community about the benefits of veterinary medicine is to get out there and get involved.

It's a fact. Your best source for new clients is referrals. Getting involved in community events says more about your practice than the flashiest brochure. What can you do for your local schools, church, and men or women's groups? Promote goodwill by providing hospital tours to groups and organizations. A new practice should sponsor an open house to introduce itself to the community. Even an established practice should open its doors every so often to let people tour the facility and see the high-quality medicine you demand.

Career days at local schools are a great way to discuss veterinary medicine opportunities available. You may not see immediate results from your involvement, but it definitely will pay back numerous dividends in the long run.

Try a three-tier reminder system

A reminder system can make or break your practice, yet too many owners pay little attention to this vital tool. A study of several hundred veterinary hospitals found that, on average, only 42 percent of patients were current on vaccinations. Twenty percent were one year past due, 15 percent were two or more years past due, and—perhaps the most disturbing result—23 percent had never received a vaccination at the hospital. In other words, your practice can estimate that nearly 60 percent of your patients aren't current with vaccinations.

Even if clients don't want yearly vaccinations, their pets still need comprehensive physical examinations. If your hospital team overlooks this vital step, you could do more than lose potential business—you could be risking patients' lives.

Remember, your reminder system is only as good as the information you give it. Do you update vaccination information when a client visits your practice? Do you get vaccination histories for patients that come in for skin, eye, or ear problems? If the client isn't sure when the pet was last vaccinated, does the receptionist ask if the pet was vaccinated within the last year? If the client says no but doesn't wish to have the pet vaccinated that day, your receptionist should note in the computer to send a vaccination reminder for the first of the following month. If the client says yes, the receptionist can ask whether it was vaccinated in the spring, summer, fall, or winter, then assign a date in the computer.

The bottom line: You need to know when the pet was last vaccinated. If you can't get an accurate date, a rough estimate is better than no date at all. In fact, I would advise that you set this rule: Do not invoice any patient until future vaccination information has been entered into the computer system. If you fail to do this, you fail to bond your clients—and you fail the patient as well.

Please remember that no computer system was designed to look up previous vaccinations. Get the information from the medical record. The reminder system was set up for one purpose: to tell clients about a preventive procedure necessary for their pet's health.

Once you have preventive health information in your computer, the next step is to set up an effective reminder system. I recommend the following three-tier reminder system:

• **Tier 1**: Send a postcard a week or two before the patient is due for the service.

• **Tier 2**: If the client doesn't respond within 30 days, send a trifold reminder letter. This is an 8-by-11-inch sheet of paper. The top shows the client's address and the bottom states the procedure. The back holds the best part: It explains to clients why the preventative procedure is so important for their pet's health.

• **Tier 3**: If the client still doesn't respond, send a "Pet Health Alert" postcard 30 days after sending the trifold letter. The postcard tells clients that it is the last reminder they will receive and reiterates the importance of the preventative procedures. I recommend that small practices send reminders once a month. Larger practices might send out reminders weekly or twice a month, but still keep the 30-day increment between each reminder.

Many computer systems let you perform a "search and sort" to find patients seen within the last week or month that have no reminder dates entered. It's a good idea to run this report weekly.

If a client hasn't responded after one year, send a "purging card." This is often a bifold postcard. The top reports that the pet is more than one year past due on preventive procedures and the bottom is a postcard that the client can detach and check off an appropriate response:

"I don't own the pet anymore," "I've chosen another veterinarian," or "I need to come in. Please call so I can schedule an appointment."

Some practices opt to phone clients instead of sending a purge card. This works well, too, as long as the team keeps a written record of the contact. Whatever protocol you use, you need an effective follow-up program for clients who are one year past due to find out what you can do to reactivate them.

Internal strategies

Client Education Tools
Some of the best marketing tools are the little things you and your staff do to further educate clients about veterinary medicine. After all, clients only buy services they know about. And if they run into a friend whose pet needs care, they'll know if you offer what they need. Here are several widely used ideas:

• **Pre-exam checklist.** Use this excellent marketing tool during out-patient office visits to track all the preventive procedures a patient might need. The form I prefer, which can be adapted for dogs, cats, birds, and any other species, lists and briefly explains each vaccination or procedure. There's also space to indicate when the patient is due for the procedure and whether the healthcare team has recommended it to the client before. (See Figure 7, page 40.)

Here's how I recommend you use the checklist:

When the receptionist pulls the medical records for the day's appointments, she completes a pre-exam checklist for each patient and inserts them into the medical records. When a client arrives, she gives the checklist to her and says, "Mrs. Smith, we've reviewed Casey's medical record and noted the vaccinations and procedures you requested for her today. We've also marked other preventive procedures we recommend. Please read this form, and Karen, Dr. Jones' exam-room assistant, will review it with you."

While the client waits for her appointment, she reads the form and becomes familiar with the procedures and prepared to discuss them with Karen. Note that I didn't suggest the receptionist review this form with the client; the exam-room assistant is best prepared to handle this task.

After reviewing your pet's health record, we have found _____ is due for the following examinations / vaccinations / lab procedures to help in maintaining a healthy life.

☐ **Comprehensive Physical Examination** Due Date _____ Recommended _____	A comprehensive physical examination is suggested on an annual basis. All pets receiving a vaccination will have a comprehensive physical examination prior to vaccination. Just as with people, a physical examination may be the most important component of an office visit, allowing the veterinarian the opportunity to completely examine your pet and discuss any medical problems noted.
☐ **Canine Distemper** Due Date _____ Recommended _____	An annual vaccination that helps protect your dog from four diseases: distemper, hepatitis, leptosporosis and parainfluenza. These four diseases are debilitating and can cause death. Nearly every dog will be exposed during its lifetime, making vaccination a must.
☐ **Parvovirus** Due Date _____ Recommended _____	A canine intestinal viral infection that results in bloody diarrhea, fever, vomiting and extreme depression. It is highly contagious and life threatening.
☐ **Coronavirus** Due Date _____ Recommended _____	A disease similar to parvovirus, but less life threatening. It is recommended that puppies be vaccinated because their immune system is not as strong as adults.
☐ **Bordetella** Due Date _____ Recommended _____	An annual vaccination given to dogs to prevent Tracheobronchitis (Kennel Cough) which is a highly contagious virus and bacterium causing a dry hacking cough that can persist for six or more weeks.
☐ **Lyme Disease** Due Date _____ Recommended _____	A bacterial disease transmitted by the deer tick which affects both humans and animals. It is a very debilitating disease to dogs. If your dog is exposed to fields of tall grass or wooded areas, you should consider vaccinations for your dog.
☐ **Rabies** Due Date _____ Recommended _____	A vaccination that is required by the state government for both dogs and cats. Vaccinations help prevent this deadly disease from being transmitted to humans.
☐ **Fecal/Stool Test** Due Date _____ Recommended _____	A stool test to detect intestinal parasites that threaten your pet's health. Regular microscopic examination of your pet's stool should be done for early detection and treatment.
☐ **Heartworm Check** Due Date _____ Recommended _____	A simple blood test done within our hospital to detect worms in your dog's heart. Heartworms are transmitted through mosquitoes and are fatal if untreated. Preventive medication is available in daily or monthly form to be given year-round.
☐ **Geriatric Blood Profile** Due Date _____ Recommended _____	Blood workup on pets eight years or older is recommended yearly to help detect many of the problems caused by aging (kidney, liver, heart, arthritis, dental, etc.). Early detection can lengthen your pet's life. Proper treatment and diet will improve your pet's quality of life. A blood sample can be drawn during an office call.
☐ **Dental Health Care** Due Date _____ Recommended _____	Tartar accumulation and pyorrhea affect most pets. Periodontal disease can lead to infection in the liver, kidneys and heart. This can best be prevented with regular dental care. Dental care starts at home by brushing or cleansing your pet's teeth with animal toothpaste or cleansing products. Ultrasonic cleaning and polishing under anesthesia is recommended as needed.

Canine

Let's say Mrs. Smith is visiting the practice for Casey's rabies vaccination, but Casey also needs a distemper/parvo vaccination, a heartworm check, and a *Bordetella* vaccination. After her discussion with Karen, Mrs. Smith will either give the green light to proceed with the additional services or she'll refuse them—and that's her right. It's then up to the doctor whether to bring up the topic again. If the client does decline a service, be sure to note her decision on the checklist.

If a client decides against a procedure, you can be assured the decision is a educated one. Note the refusal in the patient's record and list it on the invoice as a "declined service."

• **Informational handouts.** You probably already use handouts in your practice to educate clients on everything from flea control to geriatric care. These same brochures can make effective marketing tools, if they display your practice name prominently. Consider affixing foil stickers that list the practice name, doctor's name, address, and phone number to all client handouts. Why this extra attention and cost? Because you never know where those handouts will wind up. A neighbor may find it and show a friend, who could show it to someone else. Make it a rule today: Nothing—other than maybe the client or pet—leaves your practice without your name on it.

• **Senior citizen and preferred client discounts.** I'm not a big advocate of client discounts, except for senior citizens and preferred clients. I recommend you create discount cards for these special groups of clients. A "preferred client" card becomes a marketing tool when clients show the card to friends and relatives. Many practices note on the card: "This card is valid for one year from the date of last visit." This incentive encourages clients to bring in their pets promptly for annual exams and vaccinations. I generally recommend offering 10 percent off medical and surgical services.

Why offer a "preferred client" discount? The same reason airlines use frequent flyer programs. A discount rewards your best clients for their loyalty. You've heard the business axiom that says that 20 percent of clients generate 80 percent of your income. Your team needs to recognize and reward that 20 percent of clients!

Give the "preferred client" card to those who make most of your referrals or spend more than $2,000 a year with your practice. I also recommend that your staff insert an asterisk after preferred clients' names in your computer system. This system easily identifies special clients when they make an appointment. So your team can give them the extra-special attention they deserve.

Promote your senior-citizen discount by having a card professionally matted and framed, then display it at your reception desk to encourage inquiries. This prevents the embarrassment of offering the discount to a 45-year-old client. Many senior citizens live on limited budgets, so offering a discount can help your business appeal to this potential client pool.

• **Educational videos.** Many companies offer videos and even interactive CDs to help practitioners educate clients about pets' health problems and appropriate treatment. The best place for this educational tactic is in the exam room. Keep track of any videos shown in the medical record. You may even wish to loan out videos.

• **Photo mural.** A photo mural is a photographic tour of your practice. You should include pictures of laboratory, radiology, surgery, dentistry, trauma, or emergency, intensive care, boarding, and grooming. Write a short paragraph describing each area and place it near the appropriate photo.

Photo murals let clients tour your hospital without leaving the reception area. Most people never get past the exam-room doors to see the vital working areas of your hospital. Photos show them the commitment and energy behind your services.

Marketing is critical to your future success

There's no question. Marketing is good medicine and good business. And if you choose to ignore marketing, you won't properly educate clients or attract the quality of clientele you want to serve. Further, uneducated clients will likely choose inferior products or services because they don't understand the difference. Don't be afraid to get your name in the public's eye. You'll only increase the success of your practice—and your profession.

Chapter 5

The Benefits of Taking a Full-Service Approach

The full-service gas station may be a thing of the past, but today's veterinary clients still want full service for their pets. After all, who enjoys traveling to one place for medical and surgical procedures, to another for boarding and grooming, and to a third to buy food, toys, and other supplies? Unlike a pet shop or department store, your team can offer all these products and services—and the answers to clients' pet healthcare questions. And, if you don't offer value-added services, clients may choose another practice that does. Consider offering these popular services in your practice:

Boarding services
We've all seen the guilt in clients' eyes as they drop off their pets for boarding. They draw out their good-byes and look to the healthcare team for reassurance. The better you make them feel about their decision to leave their precious pets with you, the less guilty they'll feel—and the more bonded they'll become to your practice.

Actively improving and marketing your boarding services is the first step in spreading the word that you go the extra mile for your "guests." Even if your facility holds only five dogs and five cats, you can offer creative packages that entice and reassure clients. As you read about the possibilities, keep in mind that up to *90 percent* of pet

Figure 8: Boarding form

Owner's Name _____   Pet's Name _____
Address _____   Date of Admission _____ Time _____
_____   Discharge Date _____ Time _____
Home Phone Number _____   Description of Pet _____
Business Phone Number _____   Articles Left _____

For your pet's protection, all vaccines must be current. Bordetella, a specific kennel cough vaccine, is highly recommended. Your pet must be free of internal and external parasites. If not, treatment will be done at your expense. The kennel is not responsible for any personal belongings left with your pet.

FEES

Deluxe Accommodations

Deluxe accommodations include lodging in our specially designed suites or runs suited to the size of your pet; feeding twice a day with Iams or Science Diet® products (or, if you prefer, owner-provided food). Fresh water will naturally be available at all times. Your pet's quarters are cleaned and sanitized at least twice a day. Exercise will be provided twice a day in our indoor/outdoor runs. Daily heartworm medication or vitamins brought from home will be administered. All pets are bathed prior to discharge.

Daily Rates — Deluxe Accommodations			
Cats	Per Day	**Dogs**	Per Day
☐ Feline residents	$9	☐ Canine Residents Under 25 Lbs.	$10.00
		☐ Canine Residents 26 - 50 Lbs.	$11.00
		☐ Canine Residents 51 - 75 Lbs.	$12.00
		☐ Canine Residents 76 - 100 Lbs.	$14.00
		☐ Canine Residents Over 100 Lbs.	$16.00

Daily Rates — Upgraded Accommodations			
Cats	Per Day	**Dogs**	Per Day
☐ Individual cat condo	$9	☐ Canine Suite — 30' x 30' x 2 1/2'	$10.00
☐ Duplex cat condo	$13	☐ Canine Suite — 30' x 30' x 5'	$11.00
☐ Triplex cat condo	$18	☐ Deluxe Exercise Run — 4' x 4'	$12.00
☐ Quad cat condo	$23	☐ Deluxe Exercise Run — 4' x 6'	$14.00
		☐ Deluxe Exercise Run — 4' x 10'	$16.00

- To Make Your Pet's Stay Special -
V.I.P. Services (Very Important Pet)

☐ **Tender Loving Care Package**
Cost: Additional $6.00 per day
Package Includes:
• Daily Brushings
• Three Hand Walkings or Feline Play Periods
• Special Dietary Needs
• Extra Tender Loving Care

☐ **Puppy or Kitten Package**
Cost: Additional $6.00 per day
Package Includes:
• Daily Brushings
• Three Play Sessions Per Day
• Special Puppy or Kitten Diet
• Two Additional Feedings Per Day
• Special Cleaning As Required
• Extra Tender Loving Care

Additional Special Services

You may request special services for your pet while it's in our care. Please ask the receptionist for more information. Here are a few of the additional services we provide:

☐ Nail Trim $7.00
☐ Lamb's wool rug placed in your pet's accommodations $1.00 per day
☐ Administering prescription medications $2.00 per day
☐ Special handling of aggressive or difficult pets $3.00 - $5.00 per day
☐ Individual hand walkings $2.00 per walk

Name of your veterinarian _____ Phone number _____
In case of emergency notify _____
Owner's signature _____ Date _____

When your pet returns home, please do not let him/her eat or drink excessively. This is a common mistake and often causes vomiting and diarrhea. Wait at least one hour before giving a small portion of food or water. Please call if you have any questions.

44

owners request upgraded accommodations for their pets. What other service gets that kind of compliance?

I recommend beginning your upgrades with a basic "Tender Loving Care" package. A TLC package for dogs might include two individual hand walkings per day, a lamb's wool rug placed in the pet's accommodations, attention to special dietary needs, and a bedtime snack. For cats, the package might include a play period in a feline playground, deluxe accommodations in a cat condo, and extra TLC during the day.

You can charge an additional $4 to $5 a day for the basic TLC package, which also should include a mandatory bath. There are few better advertisements for your practice than a happy, freshly bathed animal greeting its owner after its stay with you.

To go beyond the basic package, you might offer clients a choice of pet accommodations. For example, a miniature poodle's owner may want the pet to stay in a 4-by-10-foot deluxe exercise run. A cat's owner may request a duplex, triplex, or quad condominium. Clients appreciate these options because they believe that by opting for bigger and better pet housing, they're making the pet's stay less emotionally painful—for the animal as well as themselves.

The sky is the limit when it comes to even more special services. In one practice, clients select the music they want their pets to hear. In another, cats watch a video of fish swimming across the screen— and yes, they *do* watch it. The possibilities are endless.

Spread the news!
The bottom line is that many clients want value-added boarding services to make their pets' stay more comfortable. If you already provide these services but your clients don't know about them, shame on you! You could be losing potential clients to hospitals and boarding facilities that actively promote their special accommodations.

If you're not offering these services, why not? Many of the practice owners with whom I consult say that boarding amenities, which pay for themselves in a short time, are what make veterinary boarding services profitable.

Any practice can start offering value-added boarding services. Marketing them is as easy as adding them to your boarding form. (See figure 8 on page 44.) Your clients will appreciate the extra care for their pets, and your practice will benefit from extra revenue.

Grooming services

Offering grooming services can be a real boon to your practice. Busy clients seek out a practice that offers grooming so that all their pets' needs can be met in one trip. But when it comes to grooming, veterinarians either love it or hate it. Practices where grooming is successful don't have a secret weapon. They do, however, have an excellent groomer on staff. As for practices with unsuccessful grooming services, the problem can usually be traced back to one source: They have a groomer on staff.

Sometimes the biggest problem boils down to economics. Most groomers are paid about 50 percent of the income they produce. There isn't much profit in grooming when you look at the basic numbers, but there is once you realize how much a good groomer can affect your bottom line. A good groomer points out skin, eye, and ear problems to clients. This awareness prompts clients to request medical services to correct them. For every $1 generated by the groomer, your practice should gain 50 cents in medical or surgical services. Groomers recommend products and supplies, thereby supporting your retail area and generating even more practice income.

Promote your grooming service by sending reminders to clients four to six weeks after the pet has been groomed. Clients appreciate the reminder. If you don't have a computerized system that automatically sends out reminders, try to schedule the next appointment before clients leave the practice.

Puppy socialization and obedience classes

Many practices offering puppy socialization and obedience classes report great success. The classes fill up rapidly and the clients appreciate the service. Even better, these classes are great public-relations builders. Obedience and socialization classes are so popular that many doctors building new facilities designate a specific classroom area in their design.

If you want to offer this extremely popular service, I recommend you hire a professional trainer or train an experienced staff member.

Promote your service in local newspapers, pet shops, and, if your practice doesn't offer boarding services, boarding facilities. Don't forget to market the service in your practice. Hang signs in the reception area and create informational handouts. Include the handouts in your hospital folders and new-client kits. Socialization and obedience classes are excellent options for a target marketing campaign. Focus on new-puppy owners and on clients whose animals are difficult to restrain during examinations. You may even consider offering one-on-one training for older pets.

Pet adoption centers

Pet adoption centers offer triple benefits for everyone involved. This low-cost investment finds loving homes for animals that otherwise would be euthanized, builds goodwill for the practice, and educates the community about proper animal care.

Your adoption center can be as simple or elaborate as you choose. I've seen successful centers that were two or three cages in a corner and a sign that said, "Please help find homes for our four-legged friends." I've also seen adoption centers as big as 20 cages.

Most practices offering this service don't charge for the adoption but instead ask clients to pay for medical and surgical services the pet already received. Most also offer a 20-percent discount off the normal fee for an ovariohysterectomy or castration. New pet owners are happy to pay the fees and follow through with the surgery.

Retail services

Every marketing study I've seen indicates that clients want to fulfill their pets' needs under one roof. That's why many practices include a retail center in the practice. Again, how expansive this area will be depends on your facility and comfort level with selling nonmedical merchandise.

Practices that successfully incorporate retail services say their top sellers are food, parasite control products, odor-control products, grooming products, collars and leashes, toys and chews, dishes, odor-free cat boxes, kennels and crates, and books.

If you decide to try your hand at retail, it's important that you identify your "milk, butter, bread, and egg" products and disperse them throughout the area. Otherwise it's like a grocery store placing these fast-moving items on one shelf where you walk in so that you can get what you want and leave. While convenient to clients, this approach isn't conducive to building your profit center. I recommend you learn all you can about point-of-purchase displays. These displays can make great promotional tools if you follow these guidelines:

1. Location is everything. Set up the display near your payment area. Let's face it, most people are lazy. Once they finish the exam and are ready to leave, they won't go back to the reception area for a bottle of shampoo. Test your display to make sure it takes just one arm movement from shelf to counter.

This is not to say that you can't create point-of-purchase displays in the other areas. One practice created a display of dog chews and other "candies" and put it at dog's height near the exam-room exits. As clients left the room, the dogs invariably sniffed the display. Nine times out of 10, the clients bought a treat.

One other note: If you're worried about theft, considering placing the display within the receptionist's view, either directly or through mirrors. Most thieves shy away from areas with an attentive staff. And a well-designed, well-maintained point-of-purchase display offers your practice great benefits that far outweigh the risks of loss.

2. The displays must be aesthetically appealing and the products professional in nature. Does your display say, "Come look at me" or "Forget I'm here"? It should invite clients to see what you have to offer. I recommend you try a grooved wall board called Slatwell. You can attach shelves, hooks, books, baskets, or other fixtures, and it's easy to adapt to your practice's unique needs.

The items you choose for a point-of-purchase display also can influence its appeal and effectiveness. Some practices have designed a "pet boutique" filled with specialty items. It's important to review your display objectively. If you were a client, would you be tempted to buy the products?

3. Clients must be able to see and feel any items they want to buy. Locate displays where people can get up close and personal with the products, not behind glass or behind the reception counter.

4. Keep displays well stocked so clients realize they can buy items from it. For some reason, people won't buy the last of any item on the shelf. Also, keep it "front end loaded." This means that the front of the display should look full at all times even if it's not.

5. Make sure every item has a prominent price tag. This is probably the most important element. How many times have you found something you wanted while shopping, only to realize you couldn't find the price? More than likely you put the item back on the shelf instead of asking a clerk how much it cost. People don't want to hunt someone down just to ask them how much an item costs. Instead they say, "I'll get it next time." Next time rarely comes.

Use a pricing gun or bar-coded labels if your computer has this capability. If you are computerized, I recommend you purchase a two-line pricing gun. The first line lists the retail cost and the second is a computer code. This makes invoicing much easier on your staff.

I also suggest you affix all products with foil labels listing your practice name, address, and phone number. Clients who use the products you offer may talk them up to neighbors or friends. Make it easy for potential clients to find out where they can get the product for their pets.

The benefits of adopting a full-service approach

Today's clients demand full-service veterinary care. By meeting these demands, you provide clients with high-quality products and services and the knowledge behind their choices. Do you still need more convincing? How about these reasons:

• A full-service approach stabilizes your client base. How many clients leave to join a practice that offers grooming services or a variety of veterinarian-recommended pet foods? Don't give clients a reason to choose another hospital.

• A full-service approach means healthier patients. After all, the more clients know about keeping their pets healthy, the better care the pets you see receive.

• By turning wasted space into new profit centers, you're improving the efficiency of your facility. Do you have a room in your practice where you've stored records since the day you opened? How about outdated drugs and supplies? Are there one or two autoclaves that you've never gotten fixed? Board six cats in that area, use it as a client-education room, or expand your laboratory.

• Finally, a full-service approach means higher profits. You generate passive income, or money generated without the veterinarian's direct involvement. What could be better than that?

As you begin creating your retail area, remember you can't just set up a point-of-purchase display and expect it to be successful immediately. Experiment with the products you offer, get feedback from clients, and just give it some time. I'm sure your effort will pay off.

Chapter 6

Hiring a Team of "10s"

Hiring and maintaining a high-quality healthcare team requires a great commitment. In fact, if you're unwilling to invest in staff development, chances are you'll never attain your practice goals or vision. Unfortunately, most practitioners don't put enough energy into hiring and training a strong team. They end up wasting countless hours trying to fix personnel problems instead of managing their practices.

So how do you get started? The first step is to recognize an employee's potential to become a "10." A "10" employee is highly motivated, comes in each day cheerful and excited to work, completes tasks as soon as they're assigned, and is personally vested in the practice's success. In a word, a "10" employee is a joy to have in your practice. On the other end of the spectrum lies the "1" employee. You know the type. No one else would even notice if the person didn't show up for three months. You're not alone if you've hired one or two of these people in your time.

It's time to end that bad habit. There is a management philosophy called "The Concept of 10s," which says you can mold an "8" or "9" employee into a "10" but you'll never succeed with a "7," "6," or lower employee. If you are truly going to develop your practice and achieve your goals, you need "10" employees. Without doubt, the No. 1 limiting factor to your success is the quality of your employees. If you have "5" and "6" employees you will only be able to develop a "5" or "6" practice. Think about businesses that strike you as exceptional. Most likely you were impressed because of the quality of the employees in that business. This was not a quirk of fate. "10" businesses know they must have "10" employees. They invest in their employees.

Think about your present and past employees and rate them on the 1 to 10 scale. The next step is the hard but crucial one: Replace your weakest link as soon as possible, then work on weeding out the rest. Maintaining "4s", "5s," and "6s" will only lower the bar, dragging the entire staff down to that level.

Personnel directors in the nation's most successful corporations hire and fire up to six employees for every one they keep. These people recognize quality and are unwilling to accept less. Turnover, of course, can be disruptive, but it's a better option than reducing your practice's potential. To create a "10" practice, you'll need stringent hiring and training tools: job descriptions, interview strategies, evaluation techniques, and open lines of communication.

Job descriptions: Plotting your path to success

No matter how hard you try, you'll never effectively manage your staff without job descriptions. Clear outlines of duties and responsibilities hold employees accountable for their performance.

Design your job descriptions for specific positions, not people. Describe the daily duties and responsibilities for receptionists, exam-room assistants, and technicians. In most practices, a staff member plays multiple roles. Written job descriptions tell the technician filling in for a vacationing receptionist exactly what you expect. Want help? See the listing of job descriptions starting on page 160.

By developing job descriptions for every position in the hospital, you've taken the first step toward creating your "10" practice. Next step: Finding the right people to fill the positions.

Creating an applicant pool

The ultimate goal, of course, is to hire a "10" employee. It's not an easy procedure and often involves wading through a glut of applicants—but finding the one person who'll adapt to the team and share your goals is worth it. Maximize your chances of finding "10" employees by being selective about where you put employment notices.

If you're looking for an associate, your best bet will be to submit an inquiry to local veterinary schools or to place ads in national veterinary journals. The best sources for a technician are technician-school placement offices. When looking for a receptionist, I'd inquire first at a local community college that teaches medical reception skills. To find a practice manager, place an ad in the Veterinary Hospital Managers Association newsletter. When all else fails, you can either hire an employment service or place an ad in the local paper.

If you decide to use an employment agency, be aware that the fees they charge can vary substantially. Still, there are advantages: Some employment agencies offer temporary help, so you can work with a person before deciding to hire them full time. Best of all, if you don't like that person you can request someone else. The agency does all the initial screening and interviewing for you.

If you opt to place an ad in the newspaper, remember that the better the ad, the better candidate you'll get. Here's one approach:

Veterinary hospital seeking a full-time receptionist. Applicant must be willing to work long hours and know how to deal with difficult people. Our hospital is very busy and requires staff members that have a lot of energy and patience. Salary is above minimum wage, some benefits. Please contact ...

Now consider this ad:

A high-quality veterinary hospital located in beautiful Central City is seeking a highly motivated, people-oriented receptionist to complement our reception team. Applicant must have at least two years' previous experience as a veterinary receptionist. Duties include client contact, data entry, telephone contact, filing and assisting the health-care team. Salary commensurate with abilities; we also offer excellent benefits. If you are interested in a career working in a great environment, please contact ...

Do you think there will be some differences in the responses you'd get from these two ads? You bet there would be! It's kind of like fish-ing: If you know what kind of fish you want to catch, you know the right bait to use. The same applies for placing an employment ad. The more specific you are, the better chance you have of landing high-quality applicants and finding "10" employees.

I know one veterinary practice whose team wanted a "10" associate so badly that they produced a professional videotape to show prospective employees the practice and explain its philosophy. They sent the tape to every veterinary school in the country. Guess what, they hired a "10"!

The three-step process for successful interviewing

You've put the word out that you're searching for a new team player, and the applications are rolling in. Now it's time to decide who you want to interview. I've found that a three-step interview process provides your best chance for success and makes the weeding-out process much less painful.

First, pitch applications that don't meet your requirements, including those that list strong skills but are sloppy or have misspellings. You don't need someone who won't take time to fill out paperwork properly. Call the remaining applicants for an initial interview.

Step 1: The initial interview

Initial interviews are quite brief, lasting five to 10 minutes, and they're designed for one purpose: to determine if the person has "10" potential. After the interview, review each candidate's credentials and consider the impression he or she made. (See Chapter 3 to review the importance of verbal and nonverbal communication.)

Think about whether the person seemed comfortable in the interview, keeping in mind, of course, that he or she may have been nervous. Did the person make eye contact? Did he or she fidget during the interview? Do you think this is someone who could talk to clients and make them feel comfortable? Remember, every team member in the hospital acts as an ambassador for the practice and affects clients' perceptions of the care your team provides.

When you've finished this step, narrow the playing field to five qualified people and call each for a follow-up interview. (Not sure what you can ask in an interview? See Figure 9, page 55.)

Avoid these questions

Many questions that seem harmless on the surface can be discriminatory and could land you in court. To avoid potential lawsuits, check your interview questions against this list of discriminatory subjects:

- changes to the applicant's name, unless you need the information to check his or her past work records
- birthplace
- religion
- race or skin, eye, or hair color
- citizenship
- ancestry or national origin
- age or birthdate, unless you need to prove that an applicant meets legal age requirements
- the names of clubs, societies, lodges, organizations, or other social groups to which the applicant belongs
- sexual orientation, marital status, and number of dependents
- health, including all questions pertaining to physical or mental disabilities.

You also can't ask if the applicant:
- owns his or her own home
- has a driver's license
- has any addictions
- is available to work on weekends

Step 2: The follow-up interview

Before the interview, review the job description for the position you're trying to fill, so you can focus on the skills and attributes a candidate needs to meet and exceed your expectations. Plan to spend at least 20 to 30 minutes with each candidate who earns a second interview. During this time, you'll want to learn about each person's strengths and weaknesses. I recommend taking these applicants on a hospital tour so you can note their responses to your practice environment. Again, pay attention to the person's body language. Does the applicant act friendly toward team members? Is he or she affectionate with patients? Do you see any signs of fear as you walk through the kennel?

When you complete the follow-up interviews, narrow the field again to no more than two prospective employees, and check each person's references. I know it can be a challenge to get the information you need from a past employer. Almost everyone who gives references has heard a horror story about what can go wrong if you say something less than glowing, and they often avoid giving a candid opinion. However, there are ways to learn whether a person has a good track record—see the tips on page 58 for ideas—and I strongly recommend this step. I've never stopped being amazed at what I can learn from past employers. If the candidates' references check out, offer each a job tryout.

Step 3: The job tryout

A job tryout gives applicants a chance to observe the practice for one day, spending no more than eight hours on site. Don't make it mandatory unless you plan to pay every person who participates. Most often you can ask applicants to volunteer without pay, but check your state labor laws first. It may be illegal in your area. In that case, you'll need to pay each applicant who does a job tryout. This means you must put them on payroll, and even if you don't offer them the job, you must pay payroll taxes and issue a W-2 at the end of the year. If your state allows unpaid observation days, ask the applicants to sign a release form stating that you won't compensate them. (For a sample release form, see Figure 10, page 57.)

A job tryout lets applicants see the practice environment in

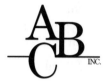

Date: _____

To: ABC Animal Hospital
1234 Main St.
Anytown, Any State 12345

I agree that I am testing for a position for employment with ABC
Animal Hospital. I will make no claim for wages or compensation for
the time that I spend in being tested for the position of employment
for ABC Animal Hospital.

Witnessed this _____ day of _____, 19___.

_____   _____
(Witness' signature)   (Applicant's signature)

Script for checking references

1. Hello, my name is (your name), (your title), at (practice name). (Name of applicant) has applied for a position on our office. May I speak with someone who can verify employment information?

2. With whom am I speaking? What's your position in the hospital?

3. (Name of applicant) states that he/she worked for your practice from (start date) to (end date). Is this information correct?

4. He/she states that the position was (job title). Is this correct?

5. He/she states that salary upon departure was (amount). Is this information correct?

6. How many days was he/she absent while employed at your practice? (If the reference is reluctant to answer this question, rephrase it as follows.) Was excessive absenteeism ever a problem with this employee?

7. Was his/her performance satisfactory? (If the reference is reluctant to answer this question, rephrase it as follows.) Was performance ever a problem with this employee?

8. How did the employee's performance compare with other employees in a similar position?

9. Did the employee supervise anyone? If so, how many staff members and what were their titles?

10. What kind of supervision did the employee receive?

11. He/she states that the reason for leaving your practice was (reason given by applicant). Is this correct?

12. Would you re-hire the employee for the same position? For another position? If not, why?

13. How well did the person get along with other employees? (If the reference is reluctant to answer this question, rephrase it as follows.) Was getting along with co-workers ever a problem?

14. Do you have any additional comments about this person's work or attitude?

15. Thank you very much for your assistance. I will keep your comments confidential.

action—and lets you see them on the job. To get the most from a try-out, team the person with an employee who does the same job. This one-on-one interaction gives the applicant a good perspective about the job and brings your team into the decision-making process.

At the end of the day, meet with the applicant. Encourage the person to share his or her impressions about the position and practice. Ask which tasks he or she feels most comfortable completing and which will require more training. Most important, ask if the job's reality met the applicant's expectations.

Before making a final decision, meet with the employees who worked with each applicant. By making your staff part of the decision-making process, you reduce the chances for "staff rejection." See, bringing a new employee on board is a lot like undergoing an organ transplant. No matter how well you want the operation to work, it won't matter if your team rejects the newcomer.

If you discover a new hire is a "6" employee in a "10's" clothing, I recommend you fire the person instead of trying to fix the problem. Remember, for your practice to reach its potential, your team members must all work efficiently together—you're only as strong as your weakest link.

Chapter 7

Training for Excellence

You might have a vision for your practice's future, but you'll never meet those goals without a well-trained, dedicated team by your side. And although almost every practice owner and manager I talk to agrees that offering team training is a vital component to practice success, a very small percentage of practices actually offer a formal training program. All too often a doctor hires someone, assigns the person a job, then is surprised when something goes wrong. Here's how you can get new hires started right and your whole team on the same page with phase-training programs, on-the-job training, off-premise training, and continuing education.

Phase training

In Chapter 6, you learned how to identify and mold a team of "10"s, and I explained the importance of using specific, task-oriented job descriptions to help make your expectation for every position clear. Now I'd like to talk about job descriptions again and how you can use them as the basis for a formal training program.

As we discussed in Chapter 6, a well-drafted job description lists all the tasks and skills a person in a particular position must master to meet the expectations for the job. The first step in setting up a phase-training program is to divide the tasks listed in the job description into three or four groups, or "phases," and assign a time frame for a new hire to learn each set of skills. Most phases can be completed in a week. Ask a star employee to train a new hire using this divided job description.

For example, say you hire a new kennel assistant. The first week, the new employee will learn to feed all boarded animals and clean their cages; assist the doctor with monitoring rounds, if needed; and clean the boarding area and runs. In Phase II, the employee will learn to get pets ready to go home. In Phase III, he or she will learn to bathe cats and dogs—and so on until he or she finishes training. (You can find complete phase-training programs for the entire hospital team starting on page 178.)

With this approach, instead of asking your team members to take on a daunting, perhaps overwhelming training job, you give both the trainer and trainee a set of clear goals and a structured program that they can start immediately. When a trainee finishes Phase 1, review the progress with your practice manager. Ask the employee to perform some of the newly learned tasks. If there's a problem at this point, you have ample time to retrain the employee before going on to the next phase.

Some practices take this concept a step further and videotape the training in progress. You don't need a movie-quality production to be effective. Just set up a camera in the corner of the reception area. Give a previous trainee's videotape to new hires so they can review the tasks they'll learn in each phase and perhaps gain some insight to ensure success.

In the future, employees can watch their videotapes to review job tasks and refresh skills. Another bonus: Use these videotapes to cross-train your staff. If you don't have a formal cross-training plan, encourage employees to start their own with the tapes.

10 recommendations for training staff

Training a team of "10s" sounds like a huge undertaking that can easily overwhelm busy practice owners. While it won't be easy to produce a team that will go the distance, you can simplify your training goals by following these 10 training guidelines:

1. Plan ahead for training. Don't let training become a "catch 'em as you can" situation. Institute a phase-training program and be judicial in its application.

2. List each subject in which the employee will be trained. Be specific. Don't just list "Customer service." Instead, divide it up into categories, for example: "telephone contact," "discharging patients," "invoicing," and "filling prescriptions."

3. List all study materials trainees must review. When appropriate, provide a copy for "homework."

4. Assign a "10" staff member to conduct training. You may use several employees, selecting those with the best qualifications to offer training in each specific area of the phase-training program.

5. Train only during your regular working hours. Trainees benefit from the hands-on experience.

6. Always set dates for beginning and completing training. Be realistic in the time frames you set. Remember Parkinson's Law: Work fits the amount of time allotted to it. By setting guidelines on how long to spend on training, you ensure the time people spend in training is focused, high-quality time.

7. Have the employee practice each new skill with the supervisor. The manager should then evaluate how effective the trainee is at the end of each week.

8. The practice owner should set aside at least one hour at the end of each week to review the training program. This is critical. Owners must be actively involved in ensuring employees are properly trained. After all, it's their business that's at stake.

9. Periodically review each employee's progress. Tell new employees how well they're doing as well as any shortcomings. Also note continuing education meetings or other education you want them to obtain to enhance performance.

10. Rate the employee during the evaluation. Be specific about other job-related skills the person needs to learn, how well he or she is doing in the areas mastered so far, and where you see a need for improvement.

Keep your team learning

Proper team development doesn't end when the phase-training program ends. Education should be an ongoing process. I recommend that you conduct in-service meetings or continuing-education meetings at least every other month. Post a notice on the employee bulletin board at the beginning of the year asking employees to suggest continuing-education topics. Then the practice manager should find someone to present the topics, either one of the practice doctors or an outside source.

Some great ideas for topics: effective flea and tick control, feline leukemia, and heartworm disease. Also consider staff training in human CPR, personal self-defense, and telephone communication skills.

Regional and national seminars and conferences are excellent sources for continuing education. State and national association meetings offer all kinds of information that's applicable to the entire hospital team. You also can find specific training seminars for receptionists, communication techniques, and technical skills. I strongly recommend you take advantage of these opportunities. If you can only afford to send one employee to a conference, ask him or her to present a one-hour seminar for the entire staff after the conference. If the employee fulfills this requirement, the practice should cover all meeting and transportation costs.

The bottom line: You need to invest in staff training if you want to build the successful practice of your dreams. Don't resort to "crisis training." Throwing people into the fire and seeing how they come out doesn't create "10" employees, only charred and scarred ones.

Other professions—including law practices, dental practices and human medical practices—spend 4 percent to 7 percent of their gross income on staff training. The average veterinary practitioner spends less than one-half percent.

If you devote time and effort to personnel development, you'll see that almost everything else comes relatively easy. A high-quality, well-trained staff can accomplish the goals you set. Without it, you might know where you want to go, but you'll never get there.

Chapter 8

Build a Team That
Can Go the Distance

Champion teams share common characteristics. Aside from boasting superlative athletes, these teams share a common desire to be the best. Members of championship teams know their roles and how they're expected to contribute to the team effort. They listen to coaches who drive them to excel, and respect each team member's contributions. Understanding the team's goals keeps players on track. And, if a team starts to falter, the coach steps in to refocus the players' energies.

You don't have to be Bear Bryant to inspire great feats from your staff. Just learn the seven basic elements of team building—vision, organization, communication, knowledge of team roles, feedback, goal-setting, and rewards—then incorporate them in your practice.

Step 1: Shared vision
It's critical that your team shares a common goal. Team-building experts agree that one way to crystallize your team's goals is to write a practice vision statement. The most effective statement is clear and concise, one that any employee can recite without having to think twice. For example:

To provide the most rewarding experience for clients, pets, and employees by satisfying the needs of each beyond their expectations.

Post your vision statement on the wall in your reception area and print it on the back of your business cards. Making it public will force your team to live up to its ideals. Once you establish a vision statement, commit yourself to it everyday, and believe in your goal. After all, if you don't think you have what it takes to get to the Super Bowl, you'll never win the Lombardi Trophy.

Step 2: Effective organization

Successful sports teams are notorious for their rigid organizational structures. Veterinary practice teams follow a similar structure. There are owners and head coaches (owners or partners), assistant coaches (practice managers and associates), and team players (support staff). Each person must know the role he or she is expected to play and conform to the authority hierarchy. You'll never see a team made up of all owners or all players.

To make the lines of authority clear in your practice, create an organizational chart that shows all team members and their relationship to each other. This chart outlines the appropriate communication channels so every team member knows at a glance who to talk to if there's a problem. If the problem is with a supervisor, the employee can discuss it with the next person up the practice ladder. A well-drafted hierarchy chart frees up the practice owner's time to concentrate on medicine and lets other team members test their management skills.

Step 3: Clear communication

A hierarchy of authority chart helps establish lines of communication for your practice, but it takes much more to guarantee open, clear communication. Make sure you're taking full advantage of these other team communication strategies.

How many staff meetings do you hold? I recommend meeting at least once a month. Larger practices may need to meet in groups— receptionists, technicians, assistants, and so on. You can have these meetings as often as you need, but still get together for a full staff meeting at least once a month.

The most productive meetings last no more than 1 1/2 hours. Prepare an agenda beforehand, listing the most important topics first.

Distribute copies of the meeting's minutes to all employees.

A staff bulletin board and employee mailboxes foster staff communication as well. Post policy changes and other pertinent information on the bulletin board. You may even ask employees to initial the notice once they read it. Make sure each employee has a mailbox to encourage interoffice communication.

It's also a good idea to require all team members to attend a communication workshop. These courses help everyone realize the importance of communication and how it affects both their professional and personal lives. Suggest this at your next staff meeting.

Other communication tools, including role playing, retreats, suggestion boxes, and staff questionnaires, also can help your team understand the importance of communication.

Step 4: Understanding each team member's role

On a successful team, players perform duties specific to their positions. Even if they know how to play other roles, when the team springs into action each person knows exactly what he or she needs to do to win. If this isn't true on your team, maybe you haven't explained clearly what you expect.

I know I've said this before, but I can't stress enough that you can't manage staff without job descriptions. To accomplish your team-building goal, your job descriptions must clearly outline the duties and responsibilities for each position. To say that your practice is too small for structured job descriptions is a poor excuse. Smaller practices in particular need this important tool. A team member may be a receptionist one day and a technician another, assuming he or she is properly trained. Simplify the strain of juggling multiple roles by telling your team what you expect from each position.

Step 5: Constructive feedback

In organized sports, athletes get immediate feedback. The crowd cheers and the team celebrates a great play. At the same time, fumbles never go unnoticed. In the days following the big game, coaches replay a videotape of the mistake so players can learn from it.

Immediate and appropriate feedback is essential to success in veterinary practice as well. Your team wants to know how well they're performing. Tell them when they've succeeded or failed. Most people don't mind being told they've done something wrong, provided you also tell them when they do something right. I often hear staff members complain that the doctor is quick to find fault but slow to praise. You must find opportunities to reinforce your team whenever possible.

Beyond day-to-day feedback, offer performance appraisals at least once a year. Quarterly reviews are even better. To be truly effective, the appraisal should be two-sided. Ask employees to fill out a self-evaluation form, telling them that you'll complete the same form. Review the evaluations together, discussing the differences. End the appraisal by recapping the positive and negative points discussed, then set a personalized goal plan for each team member. You can read more about the evaluation process in Chapter 10.

Performance appraisals are effective but make up only half the feedback picture. Employees also want to know if the team can achieve its goal. Are you meeting your vision of an excellent practice? According to the Dynamics of a Successful Practice Study, most veterinary team members don't know how well their practice is doing but want to very much. So share information with your staff. How high is your gross income this year compared to this same time last year? How many new clients have joined the practice this month? This year? How is your practice doing against the competition? How does your average income per client compare to last year? Once you share information, tap your team for ideas to improve the practice.

Step 6: Goal setting
Your team has listed goals to accomplish and enacted plans to achieve them. For example, say you want to increase the number of preanesthetic blood workups for surgical cases. Last year you had a 45 percent compliance rate. In a meeting, your staff brainstorms ways to improve this compliance rate to 60 percent within three months. They decide to create a simple but informative handout explaining anesthesia risks and the benefits of preanesthetic testing. You also design posters to hang in each exam room describing the laboratory tests and why they are so important.

To drive home the point, the team appoints a task group to write up case studies showing how preanesthetic blood workups may have saved a pet's life. Everyone acts out scenarios to hone presentation techniques and work out potential communication problems.

Each staff member knows the role he or she must play but doesn't know if the plan is working. Tell your team how close they are to the finish line by using a technique called scoreboarding. Create a graph showing the number of surgeries done each day during the three-month goal period and the percent of clients who agree to a preanesthetic blood workup. Post this in the staff lounge so that everyone can review it daily.

Think it's a silly idea? A practice I consulted with put this same plan into action. At the end of the three months, this team achieved a 71 percent compliance rate.

Step 7: A good reward system

Super Bowl winners get flashy rings and lots of money, and some even get endorsement contracts. While that's nice, the rest of us would appreciate a $100 bonus or a paid day off for a job well done.

A reward system is essential to the team-building process. After all, when your staff performs to the best of its ability, you get a successful practice, client respect, and more personal compensation. Your employees would like to know what's in it for them, too.

When your team achieves a lofty goal, I recommend you get their input before passing out rewards. Compile a list of six ideas, then let employees vote for the reward they want. Many practices opt for bonuses based on a percentage of revenue generated. You may offer to split 20 percent of the increased volume among the staff if they reach the goal.

Whatever you and your team decide, make the reward meaningful. A $5 bonus isn't an incentive when you've asked your team to devote their hearts and energies to accomplish a goal.

Foster team growth with a staff retreat

A staff retreat might prove to be the best investment you ever make in your effort to develop a cohesive team. This isn't something you can throw together on a whim. It will take some time to plan a retreat that will really impact your team.

I recommend you have your retreat on a weekend at a hotel,

resort, or private house. You may want to combine it with a fun social event, but don't invite spouses or friends unless you plan separate activities to fill their days. Some practices hold retreats each December. This lets you sum up the year and evaluate how well the team accomplished its goals. It also motivates the staff for the new year.

Once you select a date and a location, you must plan an agenda. If you have a large practice, break the team into working groups: receptionists, technicians, doctors, and so on. Appoint someone in each group to set the agenda and act as facilitator. The facilitator will ensure no one person dominates the discussion. Then prepare a retreat notebook, complete with articles for employees to read, goal-planning forms, and a written agenda.

Kick off the retreat weekend by telling your staff they have an opportunity to participate as equals in forging the practice's future. Include a review of the past year's accomplishments, comparing the practice to the previous year. If possible, list last year's goals. Commend your team for its successes and evaluate any failures.

If breaking into work groups, separate now to brainstorm improvements and set goals for the upcoming year. The only rule: Goals must be specific, measurable, and attainable within a specific time range. For example, one group may discuss how to better serve clients, while another makes plans to increase new-client numbers. The facilitator keeps the conversation on track.

Once you set goals, prepare an action plan. List those tasks it will take to accomplish the goal, then assign them to staff members. Be sure to set a time frame. Clear instructions let everyone know where the practice is headed.

Conclude the retreat on a positive note. Some practice owners share a motivational story or a movie. No matter what you choose, make sure your team knows it's vital to the practice's success.

Create a culture of empowerment

At what point during employment is a staff member most happy and motivated? I'd have to say it's the first day. It's usually a downhill slide after that, because employers tend to disempower their team members from Day 1. When employees arrive on their first day, they're excited to join a team and eager to use their skills. But more often than not, these same people are greeted with skepticism and distrust. Many new employees find they must prove themselves to employers and their co-workers before they're allowed to tackle the job they were hired to do. Even the most attentive bosses can disempower their staffs.

Consider this example. Dana, a certified veterinary technician who recently graduated from school, joins a small animal practice. She arrives on her first day excited and motivated to become a "10" employee. The practice manager meets Dana at the door, says the kennel attendant called in sick, and then asks Dana to lend a hand by cleaning kennels and bathing pets all morning. Undaunted and eager to be a team player, Dana jumps in—but she's confident she'll soon get to put her technician skills to use.

Later that day, the doctor asks Dana to assist in the exam room. As the veterinarian examines the animal, Dana notices tartar buildup on its teeth. She points out the problem to the client and explains why proper pet dental care is essential for optimum health.

Now before you continue reading, take a minute to jot down your reaction to this scenario. Be honest. How would you respond if Dana were your employee talking to your client? Now compare your response with how this veterinarian handled the situation:

After the exam, the doctor informs Dana—in front of other staff members—that it's not a technician's responsibility to discuss pet dental care with clients. Then he warns Dana to not attempt a veterinarian's job again.

Through this example, you can clearly see how the doctor and practice manager disempowered Dana during her first day. Although Dana was eager to apply her knowledge and bond with clients, she spent most of the day cleaning kennels. And when she finally got a chance to help a client, Dana was admonished instead of being commended. Worst of all, the doctor did it in front of the other employees.

Now review your response. How did you react to this scenario? Did you admire Dana's initiative and appreciate her efforts to educate a client, or did you feel a small pang of resentment that she noticed the tartar problem first? A negative reaction doesn't necessarily mean you're a bad boss. It means you're human and haven't learned how to cultivate an environment in which employees are empowered. Luckily, you can repair a disempowered environment.

You can't automatically motivate your health care team to succeed, but you can create a work environment that encourages employees to use their talents, knowledge, and experience to better themselves—and your practice. This is a culture of empowerment.

To create a practice environment that empowers employees, try adopting these strategies:

1. Provide an employee procedures manual and written job descriptions to give your team a clear understanding of job responsibilities and boundaries. (You can find job descriptions for your hospital team on page 160 and a sample hospital procedures manual on page 234.)

2. Understand that routines and rules are necessary, but don't be afraid to break them when necessary.

3. Be ready to make tough decisions, but also realize that sometimes you must reconsider your options.

4. Assert authority by achieving your high standards and expectations for superior medicine and effective organization.

5. Recognize when to introduce change and implement new procedures in a positive manner.

6. Determine what your practice must do to succeed, then help your team members accomplish these goals.

An effective manager assesses people accurately to maximize their strengths and minimize their weaknesses. Don't become so tied to the fact that you "have a policy" of who does what that it clouds your vision and hinders your team's potential.

Let's revisit Dana's first day in an empowered culture. Rob, the practice manager, welcomes Dana as she enters the practice. Before giving instructions or starting work, Rob walks Dana through the practice's orientation program. Dana receives a copy of the hospital procedures manual, her job description, her phase-training program, and a copy of the practice mission statement. Rob encourages Dana to share her skills and learn from mistakes. He stresses that the management team believes in tapping employees' strengths and making them even stronger. Dana jumps right into training, and soon she's on her way to becoming a "10" employee.

This is a perfect example of a practice culture that promotes empowerment. Think how you can duplicate this environment in your practice. But beware. It's easy to slip into bad habits, so you should make a conscious effort every day to encourage your team to excel. Changing your attitude won't happen overnight, and you may think you've wasted energy when your staff doesn't automatically respond. But keep at it. One day you'll walk through your practice doors and realize you've walked into a culture of empowerment. And you won't believe what your team can accomplish when this happens.

Start the team-building process today

Team building is not as hard as it seems. It is, however, a process that takes time. So start now to create an environment in which employees can unite their skills to reach the practice's goals.

Develop a TEAM: Together Everyone Accomplishes More.

Chapter 9

Employee Evaluations: Feedback to Grow On

One critical component of successful personnel management is the evaluation process. Effective evaluations are mandatory if you want to develop a well-informed, motivated team. If you tried evaluations and were unsuccessful in the past, try again. I firmly believe that any practice manager or hospital owner who brushes off the evaluation process is neglecting his or her business—and the people who work there.

The key to effective evaluations is to make them task-specific and individualized to the employee. You should create evaluation forms for every position in your practice: associates, receptionists, technicians, assistants, exam-room technicians, and kennel attendants. Need some help? Examples of these forms can be found starting on page 197.

But keep in mind that just because you have position-specific evaluation forms doesn't mean you "pigeonhole" employees. Like the job descriptions that were discussed in Chapter 6, evaluation forms are tools that let employees know exactly what you expect of them when they're assigned to a specific hospital area.

Evaluations also should be task specific. For example, the exam-room assistant evaluation form may ask, "On a scale of 1 to 10, with 10 being excellent, how well does the employee restrain patients in the exam room?" Task-specific questions allow for more subjective evaluations. "How effective is the employee in his or her position?" isn't as valid as "How effective is the employee at communicating preventive health care information to the client regarding his or her pet?"

Creating a successful evaluation process

A successful evaluation process involves three steps. First, it's important that you develop an effective evaluation form. Second, it's best that you give the form to the employee at the beginning of the evaluation period—not the end. This way, employees know the specific skills you'll evaluate. And this gives employees the chance to improve job performance before the actual evaluation. Third, both you and the employee should complete the evaluation form before the meeting, then meet and review each form together.

In larger practices, the supervisor typically fills out the form and then reviews it with the practice manager and owner. The owner should always have input regarding an employee's evaluation before the scheduled meeting. Once this is done, the supervisor meets with the employee to discuss the evaluation.

Remember, the meeting should be an open discussion, highlighting successes and discussing discrepancies. For example, say you rate your technician 1 for patient restraint, but she rates herself 9. She thinks she does a great job, even though a doctor was bitten last week while she was holding a patient. This is where it's critical that you discuss the discrepancy together. Both sides should know how the other is feeling and on what basis. You may find out a different employee held the dog, or your technician may realize she needs to learn new restraint techniques that minimize injuries.

Besides having an open discussion, it's important that the evaluation is fair and honest. A glowing evaluation to a mediocre employee isn't fair to you, the employee, or the practice. Most employees know if they are doing a good job or not. Often you may find employees will rate themselves lower than you will. In these cases, your evaluation might help improve your employee's self-esteem.

After discussing your ratings, complete the evaluation by reviewing successes and setting specific goals for the employee to work on until the next evaluation. Don't forget to give your employee a new form so he or she knows what to expect for the next evaluation.

The dolphin theory of management

Have you ever been to a dolphin show? If you have, you probably saw the dolphin jump out of the water, through a hoop, and back into the water again. Inquisitive minds want to know, "How did the trainers get the dolphin to do that?" Did they say, "Jump, dolphin, jump!" Of course not. They trained the dolphin to jump through the hoop.

Remember, training doesn't happen overnight. First, dolphin trainers position the hoop underwater. When the dolphin swims through it, the trainers offer a tasty reward of fish. Then trainers raise the hoop a few inches and wait for the dolphin to swim through it. Once again they give a reward for a job well done. After a lot of time and training, the dolphin learns to easily jump through a hoop high above water.

Now let's apply this concept to employees. Think of your employees as dolphins and your evaluation forms as hoops. The important point to learn is that evaluation forms should evolve right along with employees. Once employees master certain tasks, there is no reason to keep evaluating those criteria. Instead, challenge employees by listing new tasks to master. Adapt the evaluation form each time until employees are successfully jumping through hoops.

How often should you perform employee evaluations?

I recommend evaluating new employees after their first 90 days of employment, then at least yearly thereafter. However, if you incorporate an incentive program based on the employee's performance and increased practice gross, you'll need to perform quarterly evaluations. Chapter 10 explains more about this motivating incentive plan.

Whatever your policy, make sure it's clearly outlined in your employee procedures manual. If you say you'll conduct annual evaluations, you must do so. A great way to demotivate your staff is to say you'll do yearly evaluations then not follow through. Believe me, employees will know to the day when they should be evaluated. When you overlook an evaluation, you give the impression that you don't consider employees important enough to waste your time evaluating them. Avoid this by programming a reminder in the computer or making a note on your calendar. Inform employees at the beginning of the month that they're due for an evaluation and schedule it then.

Evaluations are critical in a well-managed practice. As I said earlier, you're negligent if you don't evaluate your team. Management is responsible for conducting effective evaluations for all health care team members. And when done properly, evaluations can help communication lines remain open and develop "10" employees.

Chapter 10

Motivating Your Healthcare Team

How would you define motivation? Motivation is an internally generated force that makes you want to do something. The key to this definition is "internally generated." While you can't motivate somebody to do something, you can create an environment in which they can become motivated.

Of the many practices I've worked with, I invariably notice an inverse relationship between the length of employment and job satisfaction. It seems the longer employees work for a practice, the less satisfied they are. The problem is that, from Day 1, most owners and practice managers unwittingly chip away at employees' motivation until it becomes nonexistent. The five factors of motivation are fulfillment of basic needs, a healthy work environment, security, knowledge and ability to do the job, and knowledge of the practice's employee policies and procedures. These elements must be present before anyone can become motivated. If they're missing in your practice, chances are motivated employees will be too.

Remember, money isn't everything. Just look at the automobile industry. U.S. car manufacturers paid workers extremely high wages compared to foreign countries, but who produced a better car? Employees who were paid less appeared more motivated. When was the last time a big raise had a long-term positive effect on one of your

employees? When you're thinking about what will motivate your team, keep in mind that at least six factors outweigh salary:
1. Agreeable working conditions
2. Recognition
3. Fringe benefits
4. Lifestyle
5. Challenge
6. Personal fulfillment.

Money is the easiest thing for a disgruntled employee to complain about, but it's rarely the primary reason for discontent.

Motivational techniques

If you're not sure you're good at motivation, don't worry. The basic tenet of motivation is to treat employees the same way you'd want to be treated: fairly and with respect.

Probably the strongest motivator you have at your disposal is positive reinforcement, or acknowledging an employee's accomplishments. Remember, "Thank you" can have a powerful effect on anyone. Employees often tell me, "My employers are quick to find fault and slow to praise." If you fall in this category, you need to quickly reverse this habit. Determine the positive things your employees do and reinforce them. Psychology studies show that reinforced actions are more likely to reoccur. Strive to reinforce the positive and ignore the negative—unless the negative is so destructive that you have to deal with it. Your employees should be so used to hearing you say "Good job," "Thank you," and "I appreciate the hard work," that when they don't hear the words they'll wonder how they failed you.

But positive reinforcement is more than praise and a pat on the back. Such simple gifts as coupons for video rentals, gift certificates to nice restaurants, or even boxes of chocolates may have a positive effect. It's not the gift that means so much. It's the fact that you cared enough to give it in the first place. And the more personalized the gift, the more positive the effect.

Make the reward personal

Let me share a story about a former employee, Dave. He was a surgical assistant at a practice where I worked. One day a client brought in a bloated animal, and Dave took particular interest in it. He stayed through the night until 8 a.m. the next day, when he was scheduled to work again. But he didn't expect to be paid overtime. In fact, he'd taken himself off the clock at the end of his scheduled shift. I only learned about it through the grapevine.

I knew that Dave's brother in California was getting married. Dave had planned to attend but he couldn't afford the plane tickets. I made a quick phone call, then invited Dave into my office. I asked why he'd spent the night at the hospital. He said he'd punched out at 4 p.m. but wanted to stay with this patient. I told him I was pleased he took so much initiative and that he'd be paid for his time. Then, to show him my appreciation, I gave him plane tickets to California.

When I left that hospital several years later, I conducted exit interviews. During Dave's interview, I asked him why he was always a "10" employee. Dave said he enjoyed the challenges and rewards of the work environment. He also mentioned that around the time of his brother's wedding he was considering leaving the veterinary profession to pursue human ultrasound—until the day I gave him the plane tickets. He said that if an employer cared that much about him personally then he could care about the practice as well. This positive reinforcement was successful because it went above-and-beyond expectation. Remember, you set expectation levels through your actions. Once employees reach that level, you should always reinforce them appropriately.

Make the reward appropriate

Some years ago, I was discussing positive reinforcement at a national conference. Weeks later, I received a call from an irate attendee who said I didn't know what I was talking about. I found out that this veterinarian had returned to his practice after the conference and found his employees had refurbished it in his absence. They had painted the interior, polished the floors, and spruced up the place. Wanting to put his new-found motivation tips to work, he gave everybody a $100 bonus and thanked them for their hard work.

The next day you could cut the tension with a knife. Employees not only seemed to hate each other but the doctor as well. It was about this time that he called me. It turned out that only three of the six employees did the work. In fact, the others took off early. The moral to this story: For positive reinforcement to be effective, it must be appropriate.

There may be times when across-the-board reinforcement is appropriate. Once, when I had been on the road for several weeks, my staff worked harder than they ever had before to make sure all the work was done when I returned. As a reward, I told them I'd take them out to lunch.

When lunchtime rolled around, so did a stretch limousine. My surprised associates were escorted to the limo, which then took us to a mall. I handed each a $100 bill and told them there were some strings attached. First, they had to spend the money within an hour. If they didn't, I got to keep whatever was left. Second, they had to spend it on themselves, not anybody else.

It was quite entertaining. My employees frantically ran in and out of stores trying to find something. At the end of the hour everyone regrouped and did a little show and tell. They'd spent all the money, and three shoppers who'd watched our group came up and asked me for a job!

To this day, employees will show me the things they bought and ask, "When are we doing it again?" This minor reinforcement had a long-term, positive effect.

Negative reinforcement

Despite its name, negative reinforcement is by no means reinforcement. Negative reinforcement is yelling at an employee or discussing poor performance in front of co-workers. And this only has two effects: It stops the behavior, and it demotivates the employee. Only use negative reinforcement if an action risks injury to a patient or the practice.

Job enrichment

Job enrichment is an effective motivational tool that takes many forms. For example, a kennel assistant's primary responsibility may be cleaning kennels and hospital maintenance. But you can enrich his or her job by letting the person work with technicians or assist in holding a patient during treatment. You can also teach a kennel attendant how to file radiographs and medical records or perform fecal and heartworm tests.

Enrich technicians' jobs by letting them assist with such management tasks as accounts receivable or inventory control. People can become bored when a job becomes routine. It's your responsibility to make that job more exciting and interesting for the employee.

Incentive programs

There are two incentive programs that work well in a veterinary practice: targeted incentive programs and general incentive programs. A targeted incentive program selects a specific product or service, then rewards employees when they exceed a goal. For example, say you target dentistry. Your goal is to perform 60 dental prophies during February. If your technicians perform 61 or more, they earn a $100 bonus.

Although targeted incentive programs can be valuable, their effectiveness is short-lived. And another problem is they don't always involve the entire staff and can create a loss of team effort. If you only use targeted incentive programs, consider changing targets every few months and give employees something new to accomplish.

Unlike targeted incentive programs, generalized incentive programs have greater appeal because they foster team effort to accomplish practice goals. Throughout the years, I've reviewed many programs and there's only one that I wholeheartedly recommend—basing the incentive on how much gross income increases during one quarter as compared with the same quarter last year and on individual performance evaluations. Although this can be a little labor intensive, the benefits far outweigh any negatives.

In a well-established practice, you can put 10 percent of the gross increase from one quarter—as compared to the amount from same quarter the previous year—into an employee incentive fund. Each quarter, give your staff evaluation forms specific to their jobs. (Also see "Employee Evaluations: Feedback to Grow On" on page 73.) At the end of the quarter, ask employees to evaluate themselves. The owner or manager will also evaluate each employee.

Give each completed evaluation a numerical value, anywhere between 0 and 100 percent. Adjust the scores based on the number of hours the employee worked. For example, say an employee gets an

80 percent but worked 20 hours a week. You'll convert that 80 score into a 40 because the employee worked half the hours of a full-time employee. Divide the adjusted figure into the fund to determine how much each employee receives. Say you have $1,000 in the fund and two employees. One received a 60 percent score and the other received a 40. You'd give $600 to the higher scoring employee and $400 to the other.

This incentive program creates a team approach without discrimination. The kennel assistant has just as much potential to earn a great bonus as the practice manager. The program says that if employees exceed expectations, they will be appropriately rewarded.

But the downfall of this program is that it's labor intensive. I've tried modifying the program—doing evaluations every six months or once a year—but found it wasn't nearly as successful.

If you want to try this incentive program, remember to follow the precepts. Do evaluations and reward bonuses quarterly. You can also consider this negative to be a positive. It forces management to let employees know how they measure up to your standards.

If in one quarter you don't increase gross, you should still complete the evaluations and tell your staff what they need to do to improve. Also, offer the incentive only to those employees who were employed the entire three months.

You should also use the scoreboarding technique that was discussed in Chapter 8. Employees need to know the "score" so they can help make the team successful.

More motivation tips that work

If you don't want to establish an incentive program, there are other ways to motivate your team. Here are some inexpensive things you can do to bolster morale:

1. Send a letter of accommodation for exceptional performance.
2. Buy lunch for the staff after a busy week or before a holiday.
3. Provide fresh fruit or veggies for a snack.
4. Buy flowers for an employee who's celebrating a special occasion.
5. Send birthday cards to all staff members.
6. Invite all employees to each hospital event.
7. Write "Thank you," "Great work this week," or "Thanks for all

your help" on payroll checks.

8. Work side by side with employees to better understand the complexity of their work.

9. Personally introduce all new employees to each staff member, doctor, and even your hospital dog or cat.

10. Start the day on a positive note by greeting each staff member, then end it by thanking them for their hard work.

11. Send cards to employees on their employment anniversary.

12. Hold morale-building meetings to celebrate practice successes.

13. Reward staff members who have perfect attendance records.

14. Buy a vase for your assistant's desk or the reception desk and periodically surprise everyone with fresh flowers.

15. Each month your new patient number exceeds an established figure, take your employees out for dinner.

16. Hold an annual staff appreciation party.

17. Give a small gift to each employee who receives a positive comment from a client.

18. Plan a staff social event and do all the cooking and serving.

19. Give a reception for each employee who retires.

20. Create an "employee of the month" or "team member of the year" display for your reception area.

Remember, motivation is an internally generated force. You can't force employees to swallow a motivation pill. You can, however, use the tips in this chapter to create an environment that fosters motivation. Remember, you have a lot of things working in your favor: a diverse environment, working with animals, and the opportunity to pursue many roles. There is challenge and excitement in your daily activities. Here are some commonly overlooked secrets to keeping staff motivated:

• Never oversell the job.
• Keep everybody informed.
• Keep communication lines open and clear.
• Keep the job challenging.
• Encourage self-improvement and create opportunities for advancement.
• Finally, make sure each employee knows exactly what you expect, and reinforce each one for exceeding those expectations.

Chapter 11

Delegation: Your Key to Success

Does this scenario sound familiar? You arrive at the practice early in the morning, check your hospitalized cases, then perform any scheduled surgeries. By 11 a.m., you've examined and treated the day's drop-off cases. You leave at noon for a leisurely two-hour lunch and start appointments again at 2 p.m. You're home by 6 p.m. to enjoy dinner with your family.

The truth is, this is more fantasy than reality for most veterinarians. Now tell me if this scenario sounds more familiar: You arrive at the practice early in the morning to hear, "The technician is out sick, and the autoclave broke last night so none of the surgery packs were sterilized. Oh, Mrs. Smith called and is extremely upset that her pet was sent home without getting the bath she requested. Plus, a salesman from ABC Drug Company is waiting for you and, by the way, payroll needs to be finished by noon."

Sound overwhelming? Do you delegate most of these tasks to other team members or do you try to do everything yourself? If you do everything yourself, now is the time to examine your delegation skills. Strong delegation skills can ease the stress in your life, free up your time to focus on those tasks that only you can do, and motivate your team member by showing you believe they're capable. Delegation is key—your sanity and your practice's success depend on it.

Why do people fail at delegation?

There are many reasons why doctors and managers fear delegating tasks to others. They assume no one can do the job as well as they can, they dislike change, or they demand perfectionism. While valid, these reasons are just self-defeating excuses that can lead only to frustration and failure in accomplishing goals.

If you believe no one else can do the job as well as you can, then you lack confidence in your staff. You may need to make some personnel changes to find competent employees, but the biggest problem is more likely you. You probably don't know how to delegate effectively. Believe me, I know. I used to be this way.

If you just dislike change, you've written a prescription for failure. Without question, change is the essence of success. Everything—and everyone— must change sooner or later.

Perfectionism is another matter. There's nothing wrong with it—as long as you constantly ask, "Do the ends justify the means?" For example, I know one doctor who's been working on his hospital brochure for seven years. He knows the value of a good hospital brochures. But he keeps sending me "proof" copies that he says aren't quite good enough. One day I expect to receive a brochure from him, and I'm sure it will be good. I'm also sure it won't be as perfect as he desires. But here's where perfectionism hurts his practice. How many opportunities did he miss to forge new client relationships during these seven years without a brochure? How many clients could have learned more about his practice? He could have developed a good brochure years ago to at least have on hand while he improved the "final" version.

The golden rules of delegation

Not sure you can delegate certain responsibilities? The bottom line is that you must learn to effectively delegate. Believe it or not, learning to delegate isn't that hard. Just follow these rules:

1. Make sure the employee has the ability to do the job.
2. Choose an employee who is interested in the job.
3. Clearly explain to the employee what you want completed.
4. Let the delegated project become the employee's project.

5. Provide adequate support and reference material.

6. Define and state the authority necessary to do the job.

7. Establish an adequate timetable to complete the job.

8. Institute automatic feedback controls to track performance.

9. Remember that delegation is not abdication. Regularly check in with the employee to make sure the task is being completed. Ask if he or she has any questions.

10. Never undermine a delegated responsibility.

11. Use positive reinforcement. Show your appreciation while the task is in progress, and especially once it's completed.

Now that you know the rules, it's important that you abide by them. This by far is the toughest part of learning to delegate. I suggest that managers who want to improve delegation skills choose one project or area of management to delegate. All too often a doctor tries giving up too much too fast and ends up feeling negative effects. Just like when learning to walk, you must take small steps to master a new skill.

Next, map out an action plan for how you can delegate the project and check it against the rules. Once you've successfully delegated one task, you'll find it easier to delegate more responsibilities to others. Nearly everyone on your team can have tasks delegated to them. Large practices may have a designated practice manager or hospital administrator, but even the smallest staff likely has a receptionist who handles inventory control or accounts payable. These are the first people you can choose to assume new duties.

Another option is delegating outside the practice. The harried doctor at the beginning of the chapter could have hired a service to process payroll, do quarterly returns, and prepare year-end W-2s. Other outside agencies, such as employment and maintenance services, can lessen the owner's workload.

Involving your team in the decision-making process

As you hone your delegation skills, keep in mind that you can't just dump projects on staff members. Say you return from a continuing-education seminar and are ready to incorporate effective inventory control. Fired up and eager to practice your delegation skills, you reiterate all that you learned about inventory control to your employees and ask them to implement an effective system. Barraged by information, your team politely acknowledges your suggestion and then slips away, hoping that after a week or two you'll forget all about the idea.

The first rule you need to follow: Don't suggest a new project unless you are willing to follow through with its implementation. You can't make a decision, then dump the responsibility of making it happen on your staff.

A more effective way of incorporating a new project is to involve employees in the decision-making process. First, discuss your idea with an employee and ask if he or she would be interested in helping. If the employee is interested, provide him or her with reference material. Set up another meeting to discuss what the employee learned, then together develop an action plan. Give the employee the necessary authority to do the job. Your employee takes ownership of the task, which means a greater chance of a successful outcome.

Look at the big picture

How are your management skills? Are you an effective manager or a grudge manager? Not sure? Here's how to tell the difference:

Although effective managers understand that rules and routines are necessary, they aren't afraid to break them for a positive change. They assert authority by demonstrating superior abilities that set an example for others. Effective managers can determine what must be done without a superior's input and know how to help employees achieve it. Chances are these managers already know how to successfully delegate.

Grudge managers, on the other hand, spend their day looking over shoulders and double-checking everything. They can't plan the practice's future growth, develop profit centers, or practice progressive management because they're constantly putting out fires. Learning to delegate is difficult for these managers, but they can be taught.

I encourage you to evaluate your delegation skills. Look at your routine and the success of your practice. If you're already good at delegation, teach another person the skill. If you're lacking, make learning delegation a top priority. Your future success depends on it.

What's your leadership style?

Your style can either turn on or turn off your team members—and dramatically affect their performance. The five main leadership styles, according to social psychologist John D. Lawson, are:

• **The Absolute Dictator.** Usually very able. Has strong opinions about what should be done and how to do it. Probably started practice with no help from others. Makes all the decisions. Rarely delegates anything. Aggressively cracks the whip, orders others around, and criticizes others in public. Staff feels left out, put down, unworthy, and apathetic. Some become irritated and quit. Little loyalty or enthusiasm is generated. The dictator usually works on projects alone and attracts only fearful followers or those who can't think for themselves.

• **The Benevolent Leader.** Dominated by a need to be loved and to be considered a "nice guy." Publicly praises even the smallest accomplishments. The staff is very fond of the Benevolent Leader because he adopts their every idea and attends to all their needs. Usually winds up doing the dirty work involved in most important projects, because he doesn't want to trouble his staff with it. His inability to delegate anything but the easiest tasks to his subordinates prevents him from making progress in his practice.

• **The Unpredictable Leader.** Moody, unstable. May be a dictator one day and benevolent the next, depending on circumstances over which the staff has little control. Much of staff's time is spent trying to figure out the unpredictable moods.

• **The Responsibility Avoider.** Lacks self-confidence and/or ambition. Lets his practice drift without providing direction. Employees who want to accomplish things for themselves and the practice will resent this lack of direction and usually will leave.

• **The Democratic Leader.** Listens to associates and subordinates and involves them in decision-making. Communicates openly and keeps others informed. Welcomes suggestions and takes initiative to get things done. Good at building team spirit and loyalty to the organization.

Chapter 12

When an Employee Doesn't Meet Expectations

Unfortunately, not all employees are perfect "10s," even despite your best efforts to train them. Perhaps the most difficult aspect of owning a business is firing an employee. Most experienced managers admit they've discharged people only to realize the dirty deed should have been done much sooner.

I'm not sure if people in the veterinary profession are exceptionally kind-hearted or just chicken. Regardless, most veterinarians and veterinary practice managers delay firing an employee until troubles reach the critical mark—and by this time, it's had a devastating effect on a practice.

Discharging an employee can be tricky, and some business owners hesitate for fear of backlash cries of discrimination. You can protect yourself by implementing a written discipline policy. Clearly specify the protocol you'll follow if an employee's performance slides. The most common is the "three strikes and you're out" policy. For example, this type of policy might read:

When a situation arises that requires disciplinary action, the practice manager will address the problem first with a verbal warning and note the incident in the employee's file.

If a second incident occurs, the practice manager will issue a

written reprimand, placing a copy in the employee's file.
Further incidents will lead to an employee's immediate dismissal.

Once you established a policy, it's critical that you follow through. Nothing is more demotivating to a team than working with someone who gets away with actions that the rest of the staff feels should be punished. If you continually threaten discipline but rarely enforce it, you'll end up spending more time handling personnel problems than practicing medicine or managing your practice. However, by setting reasonable limits for staff members and disciplining them consistently and appropriately, you'll gain your team's respect—and you'll have more time to focus on medicine and practice management.

Try a pre-emptive strike
Many practice owners avoid termination troubles by designating themselves as "at-will" employers. With this designation, you and your employees agree that continued employment is subject to termination without prior notice. This doesn't mean you can violate discrimination or other employment laws, but it does simplify the termination process and may avoid some labor-board problems.

If you decide to declare yourself an at-will employer, you must issue a written at-will employment statement. Inform all prospective employees before hiring that you're an at-will employer. Then, once employees are hired, have them sign the statement. But if you decide to become an at-will employer down the road, you can't force those staff members who've been working for you to sign if they refuse. Employment at-will laws are complicated and vary from state to state. Before implementing any plan of this nature, consult a lawyer specializing in employment law.

Keep dignity intact
When your feedback and guidance fails—and you've followed your practice's discipline policy—it's time to end your working relationship with the employee. Most employees know when they're not making the grade. And this can frustrate both you and the person. Letting an under-performing employee go might be the fairest move for you,

the person, and your staff. Just because someone isn't successful in your practice doesn't mean that he or she won't be elsewhere. This is why it's essential to be positive when terminating an employee.

Although firing someone is never easy, it's best to do this at the end of a work day. Never do it in front of other employees or clients. Call the person into your office where you can talk privately. Depending on the factors prompting the termination, you may want someone to witness the discussion. To keep the incident confidential and avoid defamation charges, the witness should be a partner, spouse, associate, or practice manager. State the problem and note that you've given verbal and written warnings. Tell the person that because he or she hasn't resolved the situation, you've decided to terminate employment.

Terminating employees is always uncomfortable, no matter the reasons behind your decision. But you can avoid any confrontation by using an assertive communication technique known as the "broken record" response. Using this technique, you simply repeat the original statement until the person you're talking with realizes you won't discuss it further. Here's a sample interaction:

"John, you were tardy again this morning. After giving you both verbal and written notices regarding this problem, I must now terminate your position with our practice."

John may offer various explanations for his tardiness. You would respond, "John, as I have said, I am terminating your position today because you were tardy this morning. You've already received verbal and written notices regarding this problem."

No matter what John says, you should repeat these response until he realizes he can't argue his way back into a job.

It's important that you don't offer additional information other than the reason for termination. Make sure you don't go off on tangents, talk about other employees, or bring up situations irrelevant to the employee's termination. The broken record response keeps you focused during this awkward ordeal.

Turn the negative into a positive

Although firing an employee is not an enjoyable experience, the act can have a positive impact. Firing a staff member often yields a great opportunity for you to improve your practice. To accomplish this most effectively, conduct exit interviews with all employees who leave your practice—no matter the situation. In some instances, this just might be the most important interview you ever perform.

When an employee leaves on good terms, request an exit interview before the last day. But when interviewing a fired employee, wait a few weeks before calling. A neutral environment, such as a restaurant or coffee shop, works best. Tell the person that the interview is an opportunity for him or her to give feedback about the practice, its environment, and management. Questions you might ask include:

1. What are your overall impressions of the practice?
2. What level of service and care do you think we provide?
3. Do you feel you were treated fairly by your co-workers and the practice management?
4. How can management improve the work environment?
5. How open did you feel management was to new ideas and suggestions from team member?
6. How effective was my communication and how can I improve it?
7. If you were me, what two things would you do to improve the practice?
8. If you were seeking a veterinary position in this area, would you apply to this practice? If not, why not?
9. How can the practice team improve the care and services it provides patients and clients?
10. Is there any other information you want to share?

Follow these rules: If you're considering firing someone, you probably should have done it months ago. If you're on the fence, you should evaluate the situation, make sure you haven't violated labor laws, and take the termination plunge. Besides, chances are it's long overdue. Don't brush off the exit interview, either. While these information-gaining tools are not always enjoyable, they are always worthwhile. Don't become defensive with a person's answers. Remember, you want him or her to be brutally honest so that you can make the necessary changes and improve your practice—and hopefully avoid having to terminate another employee.

Chapter 13

The Role of a Practice Manager

Nearly every veterinary practice has some type of manager, whether designated or not. No matter who it is, this person falls under one of three manager categories: office manager, practice manager, or hospital administrator.

An office manager is a staff member, usually a receptionist, who has taken on such limited management responsibilities as accounts receivable, bookkeeping, personnel management, or inventory control. An office manager spends 10 percent to 20 percent of his or her time doing management duties.

A practice manager is responsible for more management duties than an office manager but isn't as involved as a hospital administrator. This person devotes 50 percent or more of his or her time to practice management.

A hospital administrator handles all practice management responsibilities outside of medicine and surgery. This person oversees inventory control, bookkeeping, accounts receivable, and such personnel issues as hiring, training, and discharging staff. A definitive difference between a hospital administrator and practice manager is that a hospital administrator would also oversee associates in areas pertaining to practice management.

Duties and responsibilities

The main areas that a manager oversees are finance and accounting, personnel, marketing and public relations, safety and OSHA regulations, inventory, client service, and equipment and facility maintenance. How much the manager handles depends on the manager category he or she falls under. Use this outline as a general job description for a practice manager:

Finance and Accounting
- Bill clients.
- Balance daily deposits.
- Reconcile bank statements.
- Make bank deposits.
- Handle returned checks.
- Handle overdue accounts.
- Establish and enforce client credit policies.
- Maintain petty cash drawer.
- Maintain chart of accounts.
- Pay taxes and other bills.
- Run reports.
- Track hospital profit and loss.
- Arrange loans and credit for hospital.
- Budgeting and long-range planning
- Maintain accurate statements and records.
- Assist in setting fees.
- Manage payroll.
- Manage employee benefit program(s).
- Manage investments.
- Contract with financial and legal professionals.

Personnel
- Recruit, interview, and hire employees.
- Handle scheduling
- Manage daily work assignments.
- Manage training and development, including safety training.
- Conduct staff meetings.
- Conduct employee performance reviews.

- Discipline and discharge employees.
- Create and update manuals and job descriptions.
- Maintain personnel files.
- Mediate internal disputes.
- Represent management in external disputes.
- Maintain employee records and forms.

Marketing and Public Relations
- Manage direct mailings.
- Manage brochure production and distribution.
- Place ads in publications.
- Post ads and information on area bulletin boards.
- Run "open house" hospital tours.
- Manage community involvement programs.
- Establish and manage internships.

Safety and OSHA
- Maintain safety manual.
- Maintain MSDS book.
- Monitor hospital for violations and dangerous situations.
- Report and document accidents.
- Maintain safety bulletin board.
- Update own knowledge of safety practices and laws.
- File OSHA, EPA, and NRC reports.
- Inspect X-ray equipment.
- Hold staff safety meetings.

Inventory
- Maintain DEA log.
- File breakage and theft reports.
- Assure security of controlled substances.
- Perform and file DEA inventory report.
- Place and track purchase orders for drugs, uniforms, etc.
- Return or dispose of expired drugs.
- Maintain computer inventory records.
- Compare invoices to statements.
- Research new products.

Client Service
- Handle client complaints.
- Respond to client questions.
- Set up and maintain new-client programs.
- Manage appointment book.
- Send referral letters.
- Monitor client retention.
- Manage get-well cards, condolences, and memorials.
- Obtain and report client feedback about service.
- Manage vaccine and checkup reminder routines.

Equipment and Facility Maintenance
- Install and maintain computer system, including peripherals.
- Monitor staff use of computer system.
- Contract for repair and maintenance of equipment, building, etc.
- Assure hospital cleanliness.
- Assure insurance coverage of hospital equipment.

The responsibilities will vary, depending on the practice and manager. Also, just because a manager is responsible for a specific area doesn't mean that he or she must physically perform that task. It just means the manager oversees the task to make sure it's done correctly. Effective managers delegate many of their duties to others and maintain feedback controls to ensure that things run smoothly.

Hierarchy of authority
It's vital for a practice to have a stated hierarchy of authority so all employees know who to turn to when they have a problem. This matter is so important that I recommend you create a hierarchy of authority chart today if you don't already have one. (See page 97 for charts showing communication lines before and after implementing a hierarchy chart.)

The hierarchy of authority chart helps employees visualize the lines of communication that should occur. If a receptionist has a problem, he or she knows with a glance at the chart to discuss it with the head receptionist. The head receptionist forwards problems that he or she can't solve to the practice manager. If the practice manager

Hierarchy of Authority Before A Manager is Hired

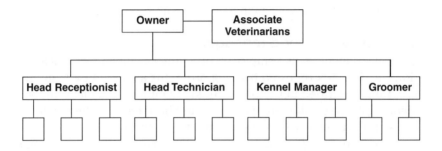

Hierarchy of Authority After A Manager is Hired

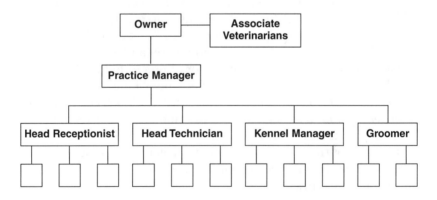

can't resolve it, he or she must then meet with the practice owner.

The chart also works in the reverse order. If the practice owner has a problem with a receptionist, he or she must talk to the practice manager, who would speak with the head receptionist, who would pass on information to the receptionist. If you circumvent the hierarchy, you undermine your management team's authority.

What makes a good manager?

Effective managers use employee procedures manuals, job descriptions, and such structured training programs as the phase training program, described in Chapter 7, to give employees a clear understanding of their job responsibilities and boundaries. They believe rules and routines are necessary but aren't afraid to break them to introduce change. A good manager knows that flexibility is crucial to ensure the best interests of the practice and staff.

If you want to be an effective leader, be ready to make tough decisions. More important, realize that sometimes your decisions need to be reconsidered. Memorize this saying: Success in introducing change is almost always synonymous with success in management.

I believe an excellent manager is one who asserts authority by demonstrating superior skills. Your technical skills and organizational sophistication will speak volumes about you and your management abilities. You must set the example for others to follow. Never ask an employee to do something you wouldn't be willing to do yourself.

Keep a finger on the pulse of your practice. Intervene and make changes without blaming anyone. Determine what needs to be done, then help your team accomplish it.

Remember, the key to successful management is assessing every team member accurately, maximizing each one's strengths, and minimizing any weaknesses.

Manager compensation

The average practice allocates 3 percent to 4 percent of gross for management. If you want to hire or promote a manager but aren't sure what you can afford, just calculate 3 percent to 4 percent of gross. If 4 percent of gross only offers $15,000 for manager compensation, you can afford to promote a staff member to office manager.

And if 3 percent of gross equals $40,000, you can hire an experienced practice manager. If your calculation nets $50,000 or more, you can afford—and more important, need—a hospital administrator to handle all management responsibilities.

It's important to realize that 3 percent to 4 percent of gross must cover all management costs. If a doctor, bookkeeper, head receptionist, or head technician spends time doing any management duties, you must factor in the cost of their time.

While most managers are paid a straight salary, some receive a percentage of practice gross, usually about 3 percent. I recommend the practice owner evaluate the manager yearly to ensure maximum effectiveness. Your practice's success depends on exceptional management skills.

Certified Veterinary Practice Manager status

The Veterinary Hospital Manager's Association Inc. created a certification program for practice managers. The program was patterned after the program that certified public accountants must pass to earn their designation. To earn the Certified Veterinary Practice Manager (CVPM) title, a manager must complete an extensive application process. If selected, the manager undergoes a three-hour written exam followed by an oral exam. Applicants must pass both exams to receive the CVPM designation and earn continuing-education credits to retain certification.

Ironically, many talented managers fail to certify because they aren't responsible for specific management areas. If you want your practice manager to become certified, make sure he or she is fully functional in all the management areas listed in this chapter.

When you hire a CVPM, you can be fairly certain you've got someone on staff who has exceptional technical and management skills. Demand for CVPMs is growing nationwide and in Europe. For more information about the accreditation program, contact the Veterinary Hospital Manager's Association Inc., 48 Howard St., Albany, NY 12207; (518) 433-8911. In England, contact the Veterinary Practice Management Association, 23 Buckingham Road, Shoreham-by-Sea, West Sussex, England BN43 5UA.

Chapter 14

Building Successful Associate Relationships

One of the most frequently asked questions I hear is, "When should I hire an associate?" Believe it or not, it's easy to answer—with a little insight into your practice's present and future needs.

First, determine why you need an associate. Is it because the practice is so busy that you can no longer handle the workload yourself? Perhaps you'd like to free up time to improve your personal life. Your answer is critical. If your practice is too busy, you face a strictly economical decision. On the other hand, if an associate means more free time, you must consider the trade-off between generating income and enhancing your personal life.

The economics of a new associate

Say you want an associate because your practice is growing rapidly. The first economic barometer you can look at is individual doctor production. Each doctor should produce between $250,000 and $350,000 before bringing another veterinarian aboard. If your numbers are lower and you still think you need an associate, evaluate the amount of work each veterinarian performs. Are doctors well supported by staff members? Do you utilize technicians and exam-room assistants? If a doctor wastes time cleaning cages, preparing fecals, labeling prescriptions, and tracking past-due accounts, you don't need another associate. You just need to leverage your staff better.

If production levels are sufficient, look at your bottom line. Say the annual cost of employing an associate is $40,000, including benefits. Can an associate generate at least $225,000 within the first year of employment so the practice can afford the additional $40,000?

The last major criteria to consider is profit-center development. Will a new doctor allow you to develop or expand profit centers? For example, an associate may mean you can extend business hours, offer exotic or avian medicine, or develop ultrasound, dentistry, cardiology, or some other specialty area. Doctors don't need board certification to develop a special area of interest. A new associate can create a new stream of revenue for you, making the initial expense a worthwhile investment.

Your financial priorities may differ, however, if you simply want to cut back on your work hours to enhance your personal life. You may want a part-time workload, more family time, or to delegate after-hours emergencies. Regardless of the reason, generating practice income isn't an issue. If this is the case, you need to consider your emotional rather than business needs.

Economically, it's simple. Can the practice afford a $40,000 to $50,000 salary without reducing the owner's salary? If not, will the owner accept a pay cut? Many would gladly say "yes" if it means more time for their personal lives. However, you don't have to settle for a pay cut. If done wisely, hiring an associate may let you develop additional profit centers. Consider your practice-building opportunities, then seek out someone who can help develop them.

How about compensation?

Some practice owners prefer paying a straight salary because it lessens competition among doctors. Yet others encourage competition and pay associates a percentage of the revenue they produce. Many associates enjoy a production-based plan because they can potentially earn more money. I prefer a hybrid plan called the Pro-Sal formula, which combines the best features of both methods.

This formula guarantees associates a base salary, but they're paid based on a production percentage. For example, say you guarantee your associate a $45,000 salary but base this on 21 percent of his or her production. To figure compensation, divide $45,000 by 24 pay periods in a year, which equals $1,875. Pay this amount on the 20th of each month.

At month's end, figure the associate's total production, then calculate 21 percent of that to determine actual earnings for the month. Subtract the $1,875 you already paid and cut a check for the balance, which is then paid on the 10th of the following month. Naturally, you'll also subtract taxes and other routine payroll deductions. If the year's total compensation falls short of the guaranteed base, you owe the associate the difference. But during my career, I've rarely seen this occur. By guaranteeing a base salary, you eliminate associates' fear of earning less. At the same time, they have an incentive to generate more income. I believe this compensation option is fairest to both associates and practice owners.

What constitutes production?

Before implementing any production-based formula, you must define production. Production equals fees a doctor generates and collects for services rendered. But there are two key factors you need to note:

1. The doctor must be personally involved in rendering the service.
2. The fees must be collected.

For example, say Mrs. Bennett brings her poodle in for a comprehensive physical exam. Dr. Martin examines the dog, administers a vaccination, and performs fecal and heartworm checks. She also sells Mrs. Bennett a bottle of shampoo. Dr. Martin receives credit for all services performed during the visit plus the product sale. A week later, Mrs. Bennett may return to buy another bottle of shampoo. But Dr. Martin would not get credit this time because she wasn't directly involved in the sale.

The exceptions are laboratory, radiology, and dentistry procedures that someone other than the doctor performs. In these cases, the doctor who requested the procedure gets the production credit. Some practices will even credit an associate with the first-time sale of a special food if the doctor discussed its use during the office visit. Also note that income derived from boarding or grooming services never constitutes production income.

When determining what constitutes a doctor's production, remember to keep it simple. The more complicated you make it, the harder it will be to track. Any inequities will even out over time. (For a sample associate employment contract, turn to page 227.)

Make the Pro-Sal formula work for you

When determining a compensation formula, follow these guidelines:

1. Keep the base realistic. If you set the goal too high, associates might not meet or exceed their guarantee. This will soon lead to feelings of disappointment and failure. But setting the goal too low isn't good either. The base may not challenge the associate, and the guaranteed paycheck will be small when compared with the production check.

To avoid these pitfalls, check the associate's previous annual production. If your associate produced $225,000 last year and you decide to pay 21 percent of production, you can guarantee a base salary of $47,250. This way, you bet that next year's production will equal or exceed last year's. With the potential for more income, your associate is sure to perform.

If you don't have a previous production figure, base the salary on the practice's income and the associate's experience. A solo practitioner can expect a new associate to generate 40 percent of last year's income from professional services.

2. Set a fair percentage. On average, associates earn 19 percent to 21 percent of their production. The percentage you pay depends on benefits and other employment costs, including health insurance, professional dues, licenses, pension or profit sharing plan, continuing education, liability insurance, and Social Security. To figure the percentage you actually pay, divide the associate's total compensation by total production. (See page 107 for a sample total-compensation statement.) Don't pay an associate more than 25 percent of his or her production unless your goal is to reduce net profits.

3. Track its effectiveness. After you've tried the program for a year, evaluate its success. By this time, associates likely are confident in their income-producing abilities and no longer need the security blanket of a guaranteed base. If so, switch to a straight production-based

plan. I've worked with more than 400 veterinary hospitals that employ several hundred associates, and the Pro-Sal formula has consistently been a win-win situation. Associates say they generate more income for themselves and the practice than they did when paid under any other compensation arrangement.

4. Determine when to increase the production percentage. This depends upon the benefits you provide. When associates receive close to 25 percent of their production (factoring in all employment costs), you don't need to increase the percentage. Instead, increases will come from enhanced competency, updates to the fee schedule, and the associate's improved ability to market products and services.

The Pro-Sal formula encourages doctors to work as a team to increase practice income. You will be surprised how eagerly an associate jumps into developing marketing strategies during slow months. One of my clients was amused when her associate asked how the practice planned to increase income during the fall and winter months. The two developed marketing programs for October and November, December and January, and February and March. As a result, the practice increased its gross income by 23 percent—and the associate earned $10,350 more than her guaranteed base that year.

The Pro-Sal formula is fair to both owners and associates. More important, new graduates want it. When I speak with veterinary students across the country, I ask them how they'd like to be paid. Nearly 95 percent prefer a combination of salary and production-based income. If students welcome the Pro-Sal formula, perhaps owners need to embrace it as well.

Help associates reach their potential

Once you hire an associate, you want him or her to succeed. Several tools can help you accomplish this. First, implement a formal orientation program. As soon as you offer a doctor the job, give him or her copies of all hospital policies, protocols, and procedures, as well as an employment contract to review and sign. On the first day, the owner should take the associate on a tour through the hospital, introducing him or her to all employees. It's also a good idea for the associate to observe various hospital departments to see how the reception, medical and surgical, boarding, and grooming areas work.

A senior veterinarian should oversee the orientation. Have the new associate shadow that person for a week or two until he or she is familiar with the hospital's protocols and procedures.

Once the orientation is done, however, don't just throw the new associate to the wolves. It always amazes me that veterinarians have no problem discussing a surgical case or reviewing a radiograph with each other but few sit in on another doctor's office visit. Where do you make or break a practice? In the exam room. Have a new associate observe other doctors' exam-room techniques and communication strategies. This can be a wonderful educational experience. I recommend that all veterinarians periodically spend time with other doctors to assess their exam-room skills.

Another excellent tool to help associates attain their potential is a production report. Most computer programs can print a report at month's end that lists the total income generated by each doctor as well as a breakdown by income types.

For example, say one veterinarian generated $3,000 of laboratory income while another billed $1,000. Glance at the production report to find out what services each doctor performed. You note that the doctor who generated $3,000 performed several skin scrapings and ear cytologies. The other did few if any. After discussing the results with each doctor, you find the second associate merely sent home medication without completing any diagnostic workup. Now the associate realizes how to better utilize the in-house laboratory.

Production reports help you increase income and decipher the standards of care occurring within the practice. Review them on a monthly or quarterly basis.

Finally, it's critical that you regularly evaluate associates on an annual basis at minimum. Associates want feedback on their performance. Design a special evaluation form just for associates (See page 200.) As part of the process, have the associate evaluate himself or herself using this form as well. Once completed, review the two evaluations together. Acknowledge all successes and discuss any discrepancies, then set goals for the upcoming year.

Evaluations don't have to be difficult or negative. They do, however, need to be done. If not, you'll hinder your employee's—and practice's—potential growth.

Keep your associates happy

I would say that the main reason associates become dissatisfied is ineffective communication. Many times a practice owner will hire an associate, then let that individual fend for himself or herself. Thus, some associates feel they're unrespected, second-rate citizens.

To ward off this monster, I recommend monthly doctor meetings. Structure these just as you would a staff meeting, preparing an agenda beforehand. You may alternate topics for the meetings, say a surgical meeting in June and management meeting in July. During medical meetings, discuss hospital policy and protocol, specific cases, or review information from a journal or continuing-education seminar. Devote business meetings to fees, business policies, and production reports.

Another way to keep associates motivated is to offer them a "piece of the pie." Before doing so, work with an associate at least three to five years. A buy-in is similar to marriage. You may even spend more time with this partner than your spouse. Let your courtship go slowly. Do you like this person? Do you respect his or her medical skills? If your associate is too eager to wait, he or she may have unrealistic expectations of what a partnership is all about.

I prefer gradual buy-ins. It not only bonds an associate to the practice but provides an exiting strategy for the senior veterinarian. You must, however, spend a great deal of time and consideration before making an offer. You'll need to draft a buy/sell agreement, employment contract, and lease between the corporation and the partnership. Buy-ins can be burdensome, but you need to keep all avenues open if you hope to retain a good associate. And forging strong associate relationships is instrumental to future success.

Total-compensation statement

This statement summarizes the various types of compensation an associate might receive. In determining total costs of employment, be sure you include the cost of all benefits. Prepare an annual total-compensation statement for each employee.

Benefits	Description	Hospital's annual cost
Wages	21% of production	$47,250
Medical Insurance	AVMA health and life	$1,440
Social Security		$3,615
Workers' compensation		$689
State unemployment insurance		$200
Federal unemployment insurance		$56
Paid vacation	on production	—
Paid holidays	on production	—
Sick leave	on production	—
Other fringe benefits	Continuing education	$500
	AVMA and state dues	$200
	State license fee	$25
	Publications	$25
Total cost of employment		$54,000
Percentage of compensation to total employee production		24%

Chapter 15

Establishing Fair and Profitable Fees

Too many practice owners base their fee schedules on competing practices' fees or what the previous owner used to charge. This becomes a serious problem when doctors and staff members lose confidence in these fees—a feeling clients can quickly sense.

Fortunately, there is a easy way you can avoid this situation and set appropriate fees. You can use a formula to determine a baseline fee for services, or the minimum amount you must charge to break even. Best of all, you can use this formula to set fair fees that will still earn you profits.

To begin, divide your services into two categories: shopped and in-hospital. Shopped services include those that pet owners shop around for competitive prices, such as vaccinations, heartworm checks, spay and neuters, and heartworm and flea-control products. These products and services should be competitively price. I suggest you call area hospitals to find out what your competition charges. Then, you can set your fees within the range and manage expenses to stay profitable.

Plus, a little insight into consumer behavior can mean the difference between a phone shopper and a new client. Say you want to buy a toaster. One store offers four models priced at $25, $35, $45, and $65. Assuming you have no information about special features, which toaster do you think most people will choose? Studies show most consumers tend to buy the $45 toaster.

This is because smart shoppers don't want the most expensive product, but they do believe they get what they pay for. Therefore, the model priced just less than the most expensive must be "the best buy."

Remember this scenario when setting your fees. Clients calling for prices on vaccinations and elective procedures have little information about your practice and may not truly understand the quality of care you provide. But pricing services near the high end tells them that you offer excellent service at a fair price.

In-hospital fees

Once you've set shopped fees, you can work on in-hospital charges. Here's where the formula comes into play. To set in-hospital charges, use this formula:

Overhead costs per minute + direct costs + return on time to the doctor

Overhead costs, for the sake of this formula, are all practice expenses minus veterinarian compensation and drug and supply costs. Pull these figures from your financial statement, then divide the number of doctor hours into overhead costs for the same time period. Divide the total by 60 to determine the overhead cost per minute.

This number represents how much it costs just to open the doors. Most practices' overhead cost per minute ranges from $1.50 to $2.

Direct costs account for all materials used in any given procedure. For example, the cost of a fecal test may include a fecalizer, cover glass, slide, and Fecasol. Once you figure your true cost, double it to cover the cost of ordering, unpacking, stocking, paying the invoice, and maintaining inventory. If you only charge to cover that true cost, you'll end up losing income.

Return on doctor time covers how much it costs to pay doctors for their skills. Large animal veterinarians may charge $80 to $90 an hour. The average small animal veterinarian can figure this return to be $120 an hour for in-house medical procedures, $2 to $3 a minute for soft tissue surgery, and $3 to $4 a minute for orthopedic or specialized surgery. Calculate surgery time from making the first incision to cutting the last suture. Consider attaching a stopwatch to the anesthesia machine to get an accurate reading. Proficient doctors can increase their per-minute charge to $5 or $6.

If you don't feel comfortable using that pricing strategy, consider this option. Use an amount based on the average time it takes to complete that procedure. This method is a fair compromise for doctors and clients. Experienced doctors still earn a fair return on their time, and clients aren't penalized if less-experienced veterinarians take longer to perform certain procedures.

Now that you've determined the figures, use the formula to create a baseline fee for any in-hospital service. For example, to establish a fee for a fecal, determine how long it takes to set up and read the fecal but don't include actual floating time. Say it takes two minutes. At a cost of $2 a minute, your overhead expense is $4. The direct costs include a fecalizer, cover glass slide, and Fecasol—likely less than $1. Now double this amount.

The return on doctor time is $0 because a technician or veterinary assistant typically perform fecals. This is true even if the veterinarian does perform a fecal. You'd have to charge for the time considering support-staff wages, which you already included in the overhead costs. Next, add overhead and direct costs to achieve $6. Your baseline, or minimum, fee for a fecal is $6, which is what it costs you to do the fecal. But if you charge $8, you earn a $2 profit.

The baseline fee formula is essential to setting fair, profitable fees. It also helps the staff understand the "why" behind the dollar amount.

Charging for pharmaceuticals

Now that you've determined where to set shopped and in-hospital fees, you need to figure out what to charge for pharmaceuticals. When figuring fees for dispensed medications, remember such factors as markup, minimum per-pill charge, pharmacy dispensing fee, and minimum prescription fee.

Although actual markup varies from practice to practice, the average is two times the cost for shopped items and two-and-a-half to three times the cost for most others. Naturally there are some items, such as Prednisolone 5 mg, that you may mark up several hundred times. Simply program all markup percentages in your computer so that each time you enter a product into inventory, it automatically is marked up.

Markups can be a problem for large animal practices that compete with feed stores and farm supply catalogs. Although the lowest markup you should use is 70 percent, you may find yourself over-priced even at this amount. If that's the case, decide whether to stop carrying those products or sell them at a loss as a "loss leader" item.

The minimum per pill charge is a default fee, depending on an item's markup. Say you set a minimum per pill charge of 10 cents or 15 cents. If a markup of two times the cost is less than 15 cents, your computer will default to the minimum charge. Most minimum per pill charges range between 10 cents and 20 cents.

A dispensing fee is an offset charge that covers prescription label-ing and preparation costs. Typically, a practice charges $6 to $12 each time a prescription is prepared and includes it as part of the total fee. Most computer systems allow you to program a dispensing fee for every inventory item. You may lower the fee to $3 to $6 for products that are only labeled and do not require counting or repackaging.

A minimum prescription fee can be charged when the total pre-scription cost doesn't equal a minimum charge. This can range from $9 to $12. Set your computer to default to this fee when dispensing and prescription fees don't meet the amount. And don't hesitate to charge this fee even though the prescription may be as small as two tranquilizers.

Outside laboratory fees
Most veterinary hospitals that use outside laboratories double the fee charged to them, plus $5. If a test is very expensive, you might only double the procedure's cost. Determining client charges in this man-ner covers the cost of obtaining the sample, submitting it to the labo-ratory, interpreting the results, and communicating that information to the client. If outside laboratory fees are calculated in this way, your laboratory should become an effective profit center.

Make your pharmacy profitable
Minimum per pill charges, dispensing fees, and minimum prescription

fees can soon turn your pharmacy into a profit center. It's important to keep track of expenses and update your computer regularly. Otherwise, you may find yourself losing money.

While you focus on building this practice area, keep in mind state regulations regarding labeling and packaging. Most states require doctors to not only label all prescriptions but package them in child-proof containers. Even if your state doesn't require it, I strongly recommend you do so. By using child-proof containers, you'll only be adding another valued service to clients.

Chapter 16

Internal Controls: Do You Throw Away Profit?

What would you say if I told you every practicing U.S. veterinarian threw $40,525 away last year? How can this happen, you ask? It's simple. Doctors didn't charge clients enough for the services they provided. It's not an issue of raising fees, it's about charging appropriately.

Do you know what's really frightening? For every dollar you don't charge a client, you actually lose about $4. That's because the services you provide come with their own expenses—your time, supplies, staff salaries, and overhead—but you don't receive any revenue. The cost of a service doesn't go away just because you don't charge a client for it.

That's why internal controls are so instrumental to your practice's bottom line. Internal controls are a system of checks and balances your staff can use to ensure clients pay for the goods and services you provide. Let's examine common problems that occur in three different practice areas—outpatient services, inpatient medical services, and the surgical suite—then implement controls to rein in the profit.

Overlooking outpatient services

Think you'd never forget to charge for a fecal? Think again. It's likely that you forgot to charge for five fecals each week last year. If you figure the average charge for a fecal is $12 and the typical doctor works 50 weeks a year, you blew $3,000 of last year's revenue.

But this is only one example. What about those forgotten nail trims? Don't let thousands of dollars slip away. The following represents a list of common services the average practitioner neglects to charge clients for each week. The high number of missed services and the total revenue lost may surprise you, but these are realistic figures for the average practice. And in larger hospitals, these figures are even higher.

1. Heartworm checks. Five missed each week at an average client charge of $22 each during a 50-week year = $5,500.

2. Outpatient clinic injections. Four missed at $12 each = $2,400

3. Nail trims. Five missed at $8.50 = $2,125

Add that to the $3,000 lost on missed fecals and you've wasted $13,025.

Do you think it's possible that each doctor in your practice is giving away that many procedures? If so, multiply your fees by the number of missed services listed here, then multiply that number by the number of doctors in your practice. That's more likely the real amount of lost revenue. Although I've said it before, I'll say it again: This is money lost by each doctor, every year.

The first step: a travel form

What if I said you could increase total income by 30 percent without increasing one fee? Whether you're a manual or computerized practice, implement a check, double-check system to ensure you charge for all services rendered. I recommend a travel form. (See Figure 15, page 115.) This form lists all procedures and services you provide and their corresponding code numbers. Have your receptionist circle the code number for those services requested by the client as well as any procedure the receptionist thinks the pet needs. Say a client complains that the pet is scooting on the floor. Your receptionist should circle "anal-gland expression" even though the client didn't specify the service.

Design your form to include several lines at the top so your receptionist can write the admitting complaint in the client's words. Attach the form to the medical record before the exam. With just a quick glance at the travel sheet, you're aware of the client's concerns and

Small Animal Treatment Sheet

Date:	Client ID:	Client Name:
Doctor:	Patient ID:	Patient Name:

Vaccinations	Laboratory	Anesthesia
Canine	455 Acth Stimulation w/Inj.	500 Anesthesia-Inhalant
145 Bordetella Booster	456 Amylase/Lipase	501 Anesthesia-Intramuscular
153 Corona First Vacc.	450 Basic Profile	502 Anesthesia-Local
155 Corona Booster	452 Basic Profile/Total T-4	503 Anesthesia-Intravenous
100 DHLP-P Temporary	453 Basic Profile/Total T-4/PQ	506 Anesthesia-Additional
101 DHLP-P #1Adult	361 Biopsy	505 Pre-Operation Sedation
102 DHLP-P Booster	438 Blood Glucose	504 Sedative
138 Parvo Booster	402 SMAC	**MSCAN**
140 Rabies Canine 1 yr.	414 SMAC-Amylase-Lipase	**Surgery**
141 Rabies Canine 3 yr.	415 Brucellosis Test	311 Abscess Surgery
Feline	433 BUN Test	300 Anal Gland Removal/Bilateral
113 FDRC Temporary	454 BUN/Creatinine	341 Anal Gland Removal/Abscess
114 FDRC#1 Adult	457 Cat Scan/Feluek	342 Aural Hematoma Canine
115 FDRC Booster	458 Cat Scan/Feluek/T-4	343 Cruciate Ligament Repair
130 Fe-Leuk First Vacc.	459 Cat Scan/Prot. Electrophoresis	344 Cyst Removal
133 Fe-Leuk Booster	401 CBC-Differencial	363 Cystotomy Canine Female
125 FIP Vacc.	460 Collection/Interpretation	335 Cystotomy Canine Male
150 Rabies Feline 1 yr.	434 Culture and Sensitivity	364 Cystotomy Feline
151 County Registration	417 Cytology	319 Declaw and Castration
Professional Services	428 ECG	320 Declaw and OVH-Feline
200 Anal Sac Expression	424 Flourescein Eye Stain	345 Tumor Removal
234 Anal Sac Infusion	404 Fecal Exam-Direct	**MSCSU**
213 Analepetic Injection	403 Fecal Exam-Flotation	**Radiology**
235 Antibiotic Injection	416 Fine Needle Aspirate	551 Barium X-ray (2 views)
239 Antispasmodic Injection	405 Fungal Culture	555 OFA Certification Fee
226 Ear Cleaning and Medicate	406 Heartworm Exam	556 Pneumocystogram/Contrast
225 Ear Crop Retaping	407 Heartworm Test-Occult	558 X-ray 10x12 (2 views)
204 Emergency Fee	435 Paracentesis	559 X-ray 10x12 Additional views
206 Examination	408 PCV	560 X-ray 14x17 (2 views)
202 Examination Re-Check	436 Post Mortem	561 X-ray 14x17 Additional views
209 Examination Multi-Patient	437 Schiotz Eye Pressure	562 X-ray 8x10 (2 views)
228 Health Certificate	440 Semen Evaluation	563 X-ray 8x10 Additional views
236 Steroid Injection	232 Shirmer Tear Test	552 IVP Injection
Hospitalization	411 Skin Scraping	**MSCRA**
605 Hospitalization	413 T-4 Total/SW Lab	**Dental**
601 Day-Patient Hospitalization	420 Thyroid Profile	755 Extract Deciduous Teeth
602 Intensive Care	449 Thyroid Stimulating s/Inj	757 Extract Teeth-Molar
674 Infusion Set	412 Urinalysis	751 Extract Teeth/Simple
524 IV Cath.	423 Urinalysis w/Sedimentation	756 Extract Teeth/Major
611 Fluids Intravenous	448 Urine Collection-Paracentesis	**MSCDE**
612 Fluids IV Additional	421 Vaginal Smear	
610 Fluids Subcutaneous	**Grooming**	
613 Fluids Su Q-Additional	866 Nail Trim	
	860 Bath and Dip	

Group Services		
1 Castration Canine	5 OVH Canine 21-50 lbs.	9 _____
2 Castration Feline	6 OVH Canine 50 lbs. Over	10 _____
3 OVH Feline	7 Dentistry	11 _____
4 OVH Canine 20 lb. or less	8 Declaw	

Cash	Check	Charge	Credit

Note: Back side of form lists medications and items dispensed.

requested services. You can choose to render whichever services you deem appropriate, then highlight those on the travel form. For multiple-doctor practices, I recommend assigning a specific highlighter color for each doctor. For those circled services you don't perform, draw a line through it. As a further check, you or an exam-room assistant should write on the upper right corner of the travel form the total number of highlighted services. Your receptionist then can compare this number to the total number of services listed on the client invoice.

This tracking system provides you with a check, double-check, and triple-check system. The check is the circling of the code number by the receptionist. The double-check is the highlight of the service provided. And the triple-check is the number in the upper right-hand corner. This form costs pennies to create and takes just minutes to fill out. I can't think of another investment that guarantees such a high return for your practice.

Omitting inpatient modical uurvioon

Is it possible that you're giving away other services each week during a 50-week work year? Consider these:

1. Injections. Four at an average charge of $12 = $2,400
2. Fluid therapy. Two liters at $18 a liter = $1,800
3. IV catheters. Three at $19 each = $2,850
4. Radiographs. Four at $22 each = $4,400
5. Laboratory procedures. Four at an average of $20 each = $4,000

And what about procedures typically considered "outpatient" that you perform on hospitalized patients: vaccinations, heartworm checks, fecal analysis, and nail trims?

The reality is that these giveaways happen too frequently. The average doctor loses $15,450 each year just on inpatient medical services. The solution is an in-hospital tracking form.

Similar to a travel form, this grid lists most routine procedures hospitalized patients receive (see Figure 16, page 117). It's more efficient than having to enter information from the travel form each day. Attach the form to a clipboard, then affix that to the patient's cage or, if you prefer, to the front of the patient's medical record. When you or your staff render any service to a patient, check it off on the tracking form under the appropriate date. This includes the examination,

PATIENT NO.	CLIENT'S NAME		PHONE NO.	ANIMAL'S NAME		REASON FOR ADMITTING	DATE ENTERED	DR.
		DATES			DATES			DATES

LABORATORY - IN HOUSE

				PROFESSIONAL SERVICES			**MEDICATION - INJECTIONS**	
Blood Screen	247			Brief Examination	3		Acepromazine Inj	1018
Major Blood Profile	209			Emergency Care	8		Amoxicillin Inj	901
PreAnesthetic	210			Examination	2		Caparsolate Inj	1411
CBC	240			Recheck Examination	5		Centrine Inj	1227
Cytology	227			New Patient Record	1		Chloroamphenicol Inj	935
Ear Swab - Mite Check	236						Dexamethasone Inj	1001
Fecal Examination	200						Droncit Inj	1237
Fungal Culture	225			**IMMUNIZATIONS**			Flocillin Inj	932
Heartworm Elisa	207			DHLP - Annual Booster	154		Gentocin Inj	920
Heartworm Test	205			Parvovirus - Annual Booster	164		Lasix Inj	1211
Leukemia Elisa Test	243			Bordetella	190		Pencillin G K Inj	934
Leukemia - FIV/Elisa	249			Rabies - Canine 1 year	172		Prednisolone Inj	1009
Parvovirus Test	252			Rabies - Canine 3 year	171		Vetalog Inj	1002
Skin Scraping	226			FVRCP - Annual Booster	182			
Urine Collection	50			Fel Leukemia - Annual Booster	178		**BOARDING**	
Vaginal Smear	241			Rabies - Feline 1 year	173		Board - Canine	395
Urinalysis	218			Rabies - Feline 3 year	174		Board - Feline	398
							Medication	394
LABORATORY - SENT OUT							Special Diet	396
Antibiotic Sensitivity	223			**MEDICAL SERVICES**				
Bacterial Culture	222			Bandage - Light	27		**BATHING**	
Fel Leukemia Antibody Test	216			Bandage - Heavy Padded	28		Bath	24
Histopathology (Biopsy)	228			Clean Ears Major	23		Clip Hair	21
Thyroid Profile	230			Clean Ears Minor	12		Comb Out Mats	20
				Clean Wound	25		Medicated Bath	22
RADIOLOGY				Corneal Stain	17		Medicated Dip	23
1 Radiograph / Interpret'n	331			Electrocardiogram	350			
2 Radiograph / Interpret'n	332			Enema	39		**HOSPITALIZATION**	
3 Radiograph / Interpret'n	333			Express Anal Glands	16		Hospitalization - Full	375
4 Radiograph / Interpret'n	334			Infuse Anal Glands	18		Hospitalization - Partial	385
				Flea Treatment	15		Convenience Stay	381
Barium Administration	320			Medical Restraining Collar	58		In Patient Medication	387
Barium Series	321			Nail Trim	14		Special Cleaning	397
Double Contrast Cystogram	323			Catheter / Empty Bladder	48		Special Diet	396
IV Urography Injection	318			Indwelling Urinary Catheter	49		Intensive Care	386
IVP Series	325			Relieve Urinary Obstruction	47		Blood Transfusion	389
Pneumocystogram	316			Splint Application	29		In Patient Evaluation - DVM	376
Positive Contrast Cysto	317			TAP Abdomen	43		In Patient Evaluation - Tech	377
Radiographic Consultation	324			TAP Thorax	45			
				Euthanasia	1896		**SURGERY - ELECTIVE**	
FLUIDS				Cremation	1897		Ovariohysterectomy - Canine	750
IV Catheter	53						Ovariohysterectomy - Lg K9	751
Jugular Catheter	54			**ANESTHESIA**			Ovariohysterectomy - Feline	752
In Patient Fluids	388			Inhalation Gas Anesthesia	400		Orchiectomy - Canine	753
Flush Catheter	105			Routine Gas Anesthesia	404		Orchiectomy - Feline	754
Replacement IV Catheter	101			Injectable Anesthesia	401		Declaw - Under 1 Year	755
Replacement IV Line	102			Sedation	403		Declaw - Over 1 Year	780
				PreAnesthetic Injection	406		Spay / Declaw	838
OPERATING ROOM				Electronic Monitoring	407		Neuter / Declaw	839
Instruments & Supplies	451			Extended Anesthetic	408			
Special Instrumentation	452						**SURGERY - NON ELECTIVE**	
Standard Operation Rm Setup	450			**DENTISTRY**			Abdominal Surgery	765
				Clean & Polish Teeth	725		Hematoma Repair	836
Medication Dispensed				Extraction _____ Min	727		Laceration Repair	759
				Minor Teeth Scaling	726		Lance and/or Drain Abscess	761
Food Dispensed				Root Canal	728		Tumor Removal	791
							COURTESY	

injections, laboratory work, IV fluids, or other treatments. I recommend the practice manager enter into the computer the information that has been noted on the form each day so he or she can review procedures and look for discrepancies.

When the manager enters the information into the computer system, he or she should compare the data posted on the tracking form to the in-hospital treatment board as well as the medical record. This way, you can be sure that all services rendered were appropriately noted on the tracking form. As the manager enters the information into the computer, he or she should circle or highlight the item to indicate that it was entered into the system as a held invoice.

When the patient is ready for discharge, the receptionist should retrieve the tracking form from the patient's cage and double check that all charges were entered. At this time, the receptionist should enter any items not highlighted then itemize and review the invoice with the client. This process also lets receptionists give up-to-date estimates to clients and compare the invoice to the original estimate to make sure the practice is charging within those bounds.

Ignoring inpatient surgical services

By now it's clear that you can lose substantial income from missed outpatient and hospital services. Unfortunately, your surgery suite has just as many problems. To avoid this, check out this list of income the average doctor loses each year:

1. Suture material. The average practice fails to charge for 3 packs of suture material each week, at an average charge of $8 a pack during a 50-week work year = $1,200

2. Additional anesthesia. Four additional hours missed each week at $24 an hour = $4,800

3. Hospitalization. Three patient days missed at $22 a day = $3,300

4. Miscellaneous materials. These include pins, plates, screws, Surgicel, Gelfoam, gauze pads, penrose drains, and so on. These average at least $55 a week. Total given away = $2,750

If these numbers even come close to the supplies given away at your hospital, add another $12,050 per doctor to your list of lost practice income.

Your operating room can be profitable instead of a big drain on

Surgical Usage Sheet

Client's Name _____   Pet's Name _____

ITEM	QUANTITY
PACKS:	
Dog Spay	_____
Cat Spay	_____
Orthopedic	_____
Other: (list packs used)	_____
_____	_____
SUTURE MATERIAL:	
Gut, chromic/taper needle	
(0, 1-0, 2-0, 3-0)	_____
Gut, chromic/cutting needle	
(0, 1-0, 2-0, 3-0)	_____
Vetafil - (0, 1-0, 2-0, 3-0)	_____
Surgical Steel	
(0,1-0, 2-0, 3-0)	_____
Wire ga: _____	_____
Hemoclips S M L	_____
Needles (not in packs)	
_____	_____
PINS, PLATES, SCREWS:	
Specify type, size & quantity	
1. _____	_____
2. _____	_____
3. _____	_____
SUCTION EQUIPMENT:	
Set up	_____
Tubes	_____
Catheters, Attachments	_____
Chest Tubes	_____
3-Way Stopcocks	_____
Other: _____	_____
ANESTHESIA:	
Atropine	_____ cc
Acepromazine maleate	_____ cc
Xylazine	_____ cc
Ketamine/Valium	_____ cc
Propofol	_____ cc
Phenobarbital	_____ cc
Gas: Flow: Time:	
O₂	_____
NO₂	_____
Isoflurane	_____
_____ _____	_____

ITEM	QUANTITY
MONITORS	
Electrocardiogram	_____
_____	_____
FLUIDS	
L.R.S. L/500 ml	_____
D-5% L/500 ml	_____
D-2 1/2% L/500 ml	_____
Normal Saline 250 ml.	_____
Blood Transfusion Set	_____
Blood	_____
CATHETERS:	
Butterfly ga: _____	_____
Sovereign ga: _____	_____
Polypropylene (fr.) ____	_____
Teflon ga: _____	_____
Tom Cat Catheter	_____
IV SETS:	
Venoset _____	_____
Travenol _____	_____
_____	_____
BANDAGE MATERIAL:	
Specify Material, Size & Quantity	
1. _____	_____
2. _____	_____
3. _____	_____
4. _____	_____
_____	_____
MISCELLANEOUS:	
Gauze Packs	_____
Abdominal Sponges	_____
Electrocautery	_____
Drains	_____
Scalpel blades	_____
Scope (broncho, procto)	_____
_____	_____
DRUGS: Injectable/Topical	
Gentamicin sulfate	_____ cc
Penicillin G procaine	_____ cc
Ampicillin	_____ cc
Lincomycin hydrochloride	_____ cc
Chloramphenicol	_____ cc
Prednisolone	_____ cc
Epinephrine	_____ cc
Doxapram hydrochloride	_____ cc
_____	_____
_____	_____

Report by: _____   Date: _____

119

your bottom line. This solution is a bit more radical than the others but no less viable. A surgical usage sheet (see Figure 17, page 119) lists all the materials you likely will use during surgery or treatment, including packs, suture materials, pins, plates, screws, suction equipment, anesthesia, monitors, fluids, catheters, IV sets, bandage material, drugs, and so on.

The form accompanies a patient into the surgery room or treatment area, and the veterinarian or surgical technician fills it out during or immediately after a procedure. Your technician or practice manager totals the cost using a master form that lists prices for the items, then he or she enters that figure into the computer or posts it on the client statement. As a side benefit, the surgical usage sheet also provides excellent documentation of the surgery. I recommend you keep it in the patient's permanent record.

Surgical usage sheets are used for nonelective procedures to make sure you effectively charge for all materials used. You likely have a priced package for such routine procedures as spays, neuters, and declaws, but some practices still fill out the surgical usage sheet to track the materials used. Typically this won't affect the cost of that procedure unless the patient was obese or over a certain age.

Many practices that use the surgical usage sheet also choose to package services that normally would be included in an operating room usage and materials charge. For example, a $25 base fee for operating room usage and materials would include one surgical pack, one pack of suture material, one pack of gauze pads, a scalpel blade, and the surgeon's cap, gloves, mask, and gown. When filling out the surgical sheet, the doctor or technician would indicate all materials used. If two packs of suture were used instead of one, he or she would add an additional fee to the $25.

If you don't charge for these materials, you greatly reduce your surgery profitability. Surgeons who charge only for their time reduce their own fee by the amount lost on uncharged materials. Don't worry about clients balking at the charge. Human medical procedures incur the same kinds of charges. Clients accept it as part of the high-quality medical care you offer.

You may be thinking, "How can I provide an accurate estimate for clients when I don't know how much material I'll use?" Good question. The answer is simple. Never give an estimate as a fixed figure. Instead, offer a range of expected fees. This way, you recoup your expenses. It's also a great education tool. Show the form to clients as you explain that they pay only for those services and materials their pet receives. Doing so will further enhance their perception of value and understanding of your services.

Reasons for ineffective charging

The causes for ineffective charging are many. We can blame much of it on overworked practitioners who don't have time to implement effective internal controls, but there are other staff-related reasons. Receptionists may not care about checking records correctly before creating the invoice. This could be a motivation problem or lack of training. You may have a confusing fee schedule or invoice system. But one reason tends to stand out above all others: You assume clients can't afford extras. You worry that they'll think the bill is too high, so you intentionally allow these giveaways.

Again, you don't need to charge more for what you do but instead charge effectively. Internal controls will help you achieve this goal.

The numbers presented in this chapter are very real. There is no question that the average veterinarian can easily give away $13,025 each year in outpatient services. Don't forget the $15,450 lost on missed hospital services, and already you're up to $28,475. Add the $12,050 lost in the surgical suite to bring us to the magic number of $40,525. Multiply this by the number of doctors in your practice.

Remember when I said that for every dollar you don't charge a client, you really lose $4? You lost $162,100 for each doctor. Is it any wonder the average veterinarian's net income is so low? Now we see why so many doctors complain they can't pay their student loans, afford the wages their staffs deserve, or take an occasional vacation.

In summary, you must effectively charge for your time, supplies, and expertise. If you want to maintain quality and excellence within your practice, you must charge fair fees, pay your staff fair wages, and earn a decent living. You've dedicated your life to offer clients the medical care their pets need. Get a fair return by implementing internal controls today.

Chapter 17

Stabilize Your Bottom Line by Controlling Inventory

The importance of inventory control has never been clearer. After the most recent U.S. recession, several leaders of Fortune 500 companies said the one thing they did to "recession proof" their business was reduce inventory. You may have heard the term "just in time inventory," which means a business stocks only the items necessary to produce the product they're making that day. Excessive inventory cuts into any business' profitability. In this chapter, we'll discuss strategies you can implement to control inventory.

Some people ask, "Isn't inventory an investment?" Remember, the definition of an investment is something that appreciates in value. What products do you purchase that appreciate in value the longer they stay on your shelves? The answer is few to none. Inventory is a means to make profit, but profits won't show up unless you generate income by using or selling goods.

A good inventory-control system ensures that you have all items you'll need for the business day while maintaining inventory at a cost-effective level. It also lets you know when to order more products. When creating your control system, don't forget these three vital components: shelf life, reorder point, and reorder quantity.

Shelf life is the time from which you receive a product to when it is completely used or sold. Say you order 24 tubes of a product, and it takes 64 days to use them up. This item's shelf life is 64 days. A realistic shelf life for any given product is one to three months. However, there are two exceptions to this rule: delayed billing and saving 40 percent or more with bulk purchasing. If you receive delayed billing, you can add those months on to the three-month shelf-life rule. If your savings exceed 40 percent, you still shouldn't exceed a six-month shelf life on that product.

The reorder point is the stock level you let inventory reach before reordering, and the reorder quantity is the amount you order once an item reaches this point. If you establish a one- to three-month shelf life for your inventory, I recommend setting your reorder point and reorder quantity at the one-month supply mark. This way, you never exceed the three-month shelf life. Naturally, you would adjust inventory to meet seasonal variations.

Computer vs. manual inventory control

Computers are a great inventory-control tool, but even the best software programs can't perform the entire job. Human error plays a big factor. You can't effectively control inventory unless all items are receipted. Although all items sold in your retail area get receipted, other items—suture material, gauze pads, syringes, and so on—don't. Some software programs allow you to link a syringe with every injection invoiced, but even these programs can't track every item.

That's why I recommend using two inventory-control systems simultaneously. Let a computer track items that go through the receipting process. For everything else, use the red flag inventory-control system. Here's how these two systems can work for you.

Computerized inventory control: When setting up an effective computerized system, the first step should be refining the category types already established in your system. Typically, these are medical, surgical, radiology, and laboratory supplies, to name a few. Delete any items that won't get invoiced, and place them in a new category titled "red flag." Next, review the reorder points and reorder quantities. Set each item for one month's usage. Most computer systems track a product's history to help you determine these numbers.

Third, print another list of items in those categories and take a physical inventory. Enter the correct stock numbers that same day.

Once a week, have an inventory-control manager create a reorder report. Any item below the reorder point will show up, making reordering a snap. When products arrive, enter such information as quantity received and amount paid into the computer. The computer will automatically update the on-hand quantity and makes any price adjustments.

Red flag inventory-control: This manual system requires more effort. Place small cards, or "flags," (see Figure 18 on page 125) at the inventory's reorder point. For example, say you decide the reorder point for gauze pads is six packages. Bind six packages together, then attach a card listing the product name, company you buy it from, reorder point, and price last paid. Place the bundle behind the rest of the stock. When you reach the bundled pack, a staff member puts the flag in a designated place. Then, once a week the inventory-control manager picks up the flags for reordering, noting the date on the flag's back to track shelf life. When the reorder quantity arrives, repeat the process—bind the products together, affix the same flag, and stock the package behind the others.

When reviewing the red flags, note the difference between the two dates, which tells you exactly how long products sit on the shelf. If this exceeds three months, you can reduce the reorder quantity. If it's less than 30 days, increase the reorder quantity.

The red flag inventory-control system is amazingly effective. In fact, some computerized practices prefer to use this system for all inventory control needs because it's simple and it works.

Effective inventory control is critical to the profitability of any business, especially a small business like a veterinary practice. Too much inventory can reduce profitability. On the other hand, constantly running out of products and supplies can frustrate and affect the quality of your patients' care.

Also, effective inventory control can shed light on any embezzlement problems. If you're concerned about embezzlement in your practice, look for these clues: income received doesn't add up to inventory costs plus markup, an item's shelf life shortens radically, or the reorder report and sales reports don't correspond. And pay par-

REORDER

THIS ITEM NOW!

ITEM NO

DESCRIPTION

COMPANY

REORDER QUANTITY

RETAIL

NOTES:

ticular attention to such items as heartworm preventive, flea-control medication, and controlled substances that have street value. Typically, these are the items people tend to steal.

To stabilize your practice's bottom line, I urge you to do a physical inventory once a year to realign product numbers. Take time today to set up an efficient system before your pocketbook suffers the effects of poor inventory management.

Chapter 18

Accounts Receivable 101

I know how hard you work for your money. But I also know you "throw it away" every time you add another dollar to the uncollected-accounts column. Think of it this way: You've already paid the expense of rendering the services, so those missing dollars represent true profit. In essence, you're taking cash out of your own pocket.

You can keep accounts receivable in check by establishing a credit and collection policy and sticking to it. The longer clients owe money, the less it's worth to you—and the less likely you are to collect it. To determine whether uncollected fees are a problem in your practice, answer these two questions:

1. What's your total accounts receivable? Small animal practice owners whose total accounts receivable are .5 percent or less of their yearly gross income deserve an A+. However, those with total accounts receivable equaling 3 percent or more of their yearly gross income have a problem.

Mixed animal or exclusively large animal practice owners should look at the ratio of their 90-days-and-older accounts to total accounts receivable. If 45 percent or more of the total accounts receivable are in the 90-days-and-older category, it's time to worry.

2. Do you have a written credit and collection policy? Those of you who failed the first question either don't have a policy in place or you're not following through. Before you can gain control of accounts receivable, you must understand and adhere to these basic rules of credit and collection. First, someone will always owe you money at one point or another. This is a cost of doing business. Second, don't spend an inordinate amount of time hunting down bad debt. Instead, develop a written policy and enforce it.

Your credit policy should include specific guidelines for team members who work at the front desk. Here's one option:

1. No client is allowed to charge any portion of his or her bill without the doctor's or practice manager's permission. Make a note on the medical record or use a colored dot to indicate clients who are routinely allowed to charge for services rendered.

2. Encourage clients to pay with cash, check, or charge cards.

3. On bills exceeding $100, clients may pay half of their bill at discharge and leave a check for the balance that will be held for up to one month. On bills in excess of $200, an additional month can be granted for an extra held check.

4. Inform clients that any bill not paid by the end of the month will incur a service charge at the rate of 1.5 percent per month, 18 percent per year, with a minimum charge of $4 per month.

5. Provide written estimates for all procedures. For first-time clients and all emergencies, a 50-percent deposit on the estimate is required.

Your practice collection policy should outline the steps your staff will take if an account remains unpaid. For example:

1. Send bills on the first of the month.

2. At 30 days, send a standard statement indicating the client's balance and the service charge assessed.

3. At 60 days, send a second statement, along with a first collection letter. (See sample letters on page 129.) Assess additional service charges.

4. At 90 days, send a third statement, along with a final collection letter. (See sample letters on this page.) Assess additional ser-

vice charges.

5. *If the client doesn't respond within 15 days of receiving the third statement, call the client to request full payment or to set up a payment plan.*

6. *If the account isn't satisfied within 15 days after the telephone conversation, review it to assess whether it is collectable. If it's deemed collectable, forward it to a qualified collection agency or collection lawyer. If the account is not deemed collectable, forward it to a qualified collection agency, then write it off.*

The following are samples of a first and a final collection letter.

Dear Client:

I am writing to you regarding your account, which is considerably delinquent at this time.

As you are well aware, all the doctors and staff at (Practice Name) strive to provide the utmost in quality care and service to our clients. It is distressing to us when our valued clients allow their accounts to age without any payment on them.

If there is a problem regarding your statement, please call our office. If not, please help retain your credit status with us and forward payment in the amount of $_____. Your help and cooperation in this matter would be greatly appreciated.

Dear Client:

Continued requests have been made by this office for you to settle your outstanding account with us. To date, you have failed to respond or indicate any type of repayment plan.

As a result, we feel that we have no alternative other than to refer your account to our attorney for collection. In addition, any future services requested by you will require full payment on your outstanding balance plus c.o.d. on current services provided.

Once we refer your account to our attorney, he will pursue collection through litigation. At that time, you will be held responsible for all attorney's fees, court costs, and costs of litigation.

We feel it is very unfortunate that we have been forced to pursue this course of action. If you wish, payment in the amount of

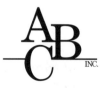

PAYMENT INSTALLMENT AGREEMENT

(DATE)

For value received and professional services rendered, I agree to pay to the order of the _____ , in the sum of _____ ($ _____). I will pay the entire sum on **or** before the _____ day of _____ , 19___ . I will pay the sum of $_____ each _____ , commencing on the _____ day of _____ , 19___ .

I do further agree that should **any** payment or the full amount of the sum stated above become overdue more than five days from the above agreed time of payment or payments, the entire balance shall be considered in default and become due and payable with service charges from the date of default at the rate of 1.5 percent per month, which is an annual percentage rate of 18 percent applied to the previous balance without deducting current payments <u>and with the addition of any or all collection agency and/or attorney fees necessary to collect the full amount due to the (Practice Name) without any relief whatever from Valuation or Appraisement Laws</u>. It is further agreed that there will be a minimum service charge of $4 per month assessed to my account while it is default.

The drawers waive presentment for payment, protest, notice of protest and non-payment of this note and agree that on default in payment of this note or any part, principal or interest, when due the whole amount remaining unpaid shall, without notice of non-payment or demand of payment, immediately become due and payable.

I certify that I have read the foregoing PAYMENT INSTALLMENT AGREEMENT and understand the terms and conditions thereof before signing below.

Signer: _____ Employment: _____

Address: _____

_____

    (City)   (State)   (Zip)

Phone No: _____

Social Security No: _____

A copy of this PAYMENT INSTALLMENT AGREEMENT will be given to the signer of the note upon request.

$_____ can be made to our office on or before _____ to avoid this process.

As you enforce credit and collection policies, take care not to punish good clients. Long-term clients who always pay on time are excellent credit candidates. You may want to check out charge cards offered exclusively to veterinary hospitals. CareCredit and Charge Guard are two companies offering credit services. Clients simply fill out an application form and, if approved, may charge up to a pre-established limit.

Tackling the problem head-on

It's easy to create credit and collection policies. The hard part is enforcing them. All practice employees, including the doctors, must adhere to the rules. If you make an exception even once, you undermine the staff's efforts and in essence void the policy.

This doesn't mean you should shut out compassion. A well-written policy makes room for those occasions when a client can't pay a costly bill. Written estimates can be crucial in these instances. When presenting the estimate, the doctor or practice manager can assess the situation. Look at the client's past payment history as well as the relationship you share. You may elect to hold a check for another month or let the client make monthly payments.

If the client doesn't follow through, consider it uncollected debt and start collection proceedings. Don't falter on this point. Look at it this way: You and your staff didn't run out into the street, grab a person who's walking a dog, drag the two into your hospital, and say, "We're going to treat this animal whether you like it or not." Pet owners come to your practice on their own. It's your job to tell them what's wrong with their pets, the necessary treatment or surgery involved, and the cost—not to assume financial responsibility for the final outcome. Clients must decide if they can pay.

If a client hesitates, you can offer a flexible payment plan (see Figure 19, page 130) or, if possible, other acceptable but less expensive treatment options. If the person is unwilling to work out a reasonable arrangement, your hands are tied. Tell your client to either make financial arrangements elsewhere or to take the pet to another veterinary facility. You must hold clients accountable for their pets' health care. If you don't, you'll never gain control of accounts receivable.

Flexibility and compassion are the secrets

Remember, you can enforce your policy and still make room for charity. In fact, I believe that veterinarians should offer free or discounted services in certain situations as a goodwill gesture to their communities. I recommend you create a charity account for each doctor in the practice. Set it up as you would a new client account, then allot hospital funds to cover fee deviations or Good Samaritan services.

For example, each doctor starts the year with a $1,000 balance in the charity account. Doctors who've depleted their funds can either borrow from another or have money deducted from their paychecks. Charity accounts offer clients flexibility and enhance community relations while keeping uncollected debt within acceptable norms.

Offering credit isn't a bad idea, provided you get paid. The challenge, of course, is deciding when you'll extend it—and when you won't. Experts agree that first-time clients and emergencies pose the greatest risk. They estimate that 80 percent to 90 percent of bad debts will originate from these two sources. Address this issue in your policy. For example, request a 50 percent or greater deposit on first-time or emergency patients. One note of caution: Beware of clients who say money is no problem. They may have no intention of paying you.

Keep in mind, clients who owe you money make up a small portion of your client base, and those who refuse to pay at all represent an even smaller portion. Don't waste valuable time and energy nagging clients who owe you money. Instead, head off problems from the start with clear credit and collection policies—and spend your time and attention providing the highest-quality service and care for the 98 percent of clients who pay.

Chapter 19

Doctor Compensation in a Partnership or Corporation

As a practice management consultant, one of the more common problems I deal with is something I call "dysfunctional partnerships." This problem can involve any number of partners who, for one reason or another, no longer see eye to eye on practice management. Often "management by objection" occurs: One partner always finds a reason to dismiss an idea the other has. Once a practice acquires dysfunctional partnership syndrome, it stagnates. If the owners don't take drastic steps to cure it, it may even go bankrupt.

A common cause for the problem is partner compensation. Many partnerships are structured so the owners receive equal compensation. This works well if the partners function equally in the practice and put in similar hours. When one partner works more or less than the other, however, tensions mount.

I recommend you establish a compensation structure by which partners are paid based on the actual work they do, a return on their investment, and a division of net profit. This system is called the "Three-Tier Compensation Program" and is used by hundreds of hospitals nationwide. You can also include a fourth tier for practice management responsibilities. If a partner handles any management duties, he or she should receive additional compensation beyond the three tiers. If one partner is responsible for all management duties, he or she should get the full amount allocated in your practice budget. Remember, you shouldn't spend more than 4 percent of gross on management costs. To set up the three-tier formula in your practice, follow these guidelines:

Tier one: Production

This first tier calculates partner compensation based on a doctor's production as outlined in Chapter 14. It's important to stipulate that the fees must be collected to count toward compensation. The average doctor receives 21 percent to 22 percent of production. You typically won't include income from boarding, grooming, and pet food sales in this tier.

To avoid confusion in defining production, the partners must establish guidelines. I recommend that a doctor be formally involved in the delivery of any service before he or she receives production credit. Exceptions to this rule are a veterinarian who orders a radiograph or laboratory procedures or schedules a dentistry. Although the veterinarian may not actually do the procedure, he or she ordered it and will supervise.

Tier two: Return on investment

Tier two involves the owners agreeing on a fair return on investment (ROI). Most practices choose 12 percent of the practice's value. You must determine practice value yearly to ensure each partner receives an appropriate ROI.

Let's say a practice's stock is valued at $500,000. One partner owns 70 percent of shares while the other owns 30. The shares of the partner with a controlling interest would be valued at $350,000 while the other's would be valued at $150,000. Paying doctors 12 percent ROI would provide annual compensation in this tier of $42,000 and $18,000, respectively.

Tier three: Division of net profit

The practice's net profit is income left after paying all accounts payable to current, including salaries and drug and supply expenses. You can divide this tier several ways. Some practices divide net profit equally among owners; others base it on the number of hours each partner worked. Another alternative—perhaps the fairest—is to use tier one. Calculate the owners' total production, then figure the percentage that each partner generated. Divide the net profit according to those same percentages. This means that if one partner was responsible for 70 percent of production income, he or she should receive 70 percent of the net profit.

Putting the formula to work

To see how this works, let's apply the formula to several scenarios:

1. Practice One has two partners. The senior partner has decided to pursue other interests and will no longer be active in the hospital. He does, however, wish to retain ownership. The junior partner will continue to work full time. In this situation, the senior partner is entitled to compensation only in tier two—ROI because he won't produce income for the practice. He should not receive production income or net profit. If the practice were valued at $525,000 and the partners agreed to pay a 12 percent ROI, the senior partner's annual compensation from the practice would be $31,500. The junior partner could earn substantially more because he is entitled to production and ROI, as well as all the net profit.

2. Practice Two is a little more complicated. In this partnership, three owners all work at the practice but are at different stages in their careers. These partners own equal shares in a practice valued at $920,000 and agreed to pay each other 21 percent of production.

Dr. Senior, who started the practice 30 years ago, now wants to work less and devote more time to other interests. He works two days a week and produces $110,000 of revenue, or 16 percent of total owner production.

Dr. Special is a board-certified surgeon who has been with the practice for five years. Although she works as a general practitioner, her goal is to develop a full-time surgical referral practice. She produces $260,000 a year, or 38 percent of total owner production.

Dr. New just joined the partnership with significant education debt. In addition to school loans, he has a mortgage and a new baby. To pay his bills, Dr. New must work extra hours. His annual production is $310,000—or 46 percent of total owner production.

At the end of the year, the practice made a profit of $32,000. Here is a breakdown of each doctor's compensation based on the formula:

Dr. Senior
Production $23,100
ROI $36,800
Division of Net Profit $5,120
TOTAL $65,020

Dr. Special
Production $54,600
ROI $36,800
Division of Net Profit $12,160
TOTAL $103,560

Dr. New
Production $65,100
ROI 36,800
Division of Net Profit $14,720
TOTAL $116,620

The three-tier compensation formula works so well because each doctor can pursue his or her individual goals yet maintain a strong partnership. Dr. Senior works fewer hours without feeling guilty and still receives a fair ROI. Dr. Special is compensated fairly for her production and ROI as she builds her referral practice. Dr. New can continue at his current pace until he pays off his loans, then may choose to cut back.

3. Here's an example of variation in ownership. Dr. Smart started his practice 15 years ago and now grosses more than $1 million. He credits his success to the fact that he invites associates to buy shares after they've been with the practice five years. Each year, the doctors can buy a predetermined number of shares.

Dr. Smart has maintained 51 percent ownership in his practice while his three partners own varying levels of interest. Dr. Rich owns 22 percent, Dr. Young owns 17 percent, and Dr. Owe owns 10 percent. The practice's stock is valued at $1.4 million. Each partner agreed to receive 20 percent of his or her production.

The partners produce the following annual revenue:
Dr. Smart $290,000 (31 percent of total owner production)
Dr. Rich $260,000 (27 percent)
Dr. Young $180,000 (19 percent)
Dr. Owe $220,000 (23 percent)

The practice showed a net profit of $52,000, and each partner will receive a 12 percent ROI. With this in mind, here's each doctor's annual compensation:

Dr. Smart
Production $58,000
ROI $85,680
Division of Net Profit $16,120
TOTAL $159,800

Dr. Rich
Production $52,000
ROI $36,960
Division of Net Profit $14,040
TOTAL $103,000

Dr. Young
Production $36,000
ROI $28,560
Division of Net Profit $9,880
TOTAL $74,440

Dr. Owe
Production $44,000
ROI $16,800
Division of Net Profit $11,960
TOTAL $72,760

Although Dr. Smart retains controlling interest in the practice, he may decide to step down and sell his shares to the other owners, either gradually or all at once. Unlike many of his colleagues who are having trouble selling their practices, Dr. Smart is preparing for his buy-out. If the selling doctor is fortunate enough to find a buyer, many times the buy-out would be on the buyer's terms, not the seller.

For example, the purchaser may choose to eliminate the seller's role in the practice and may also require a noncompete agreement stating the seller can't practice within a five-mile radius for two or more years. Cultivating an associate to gradually buy into the practice gives the selling doctor more control over his or her future with the practice.

Writing the paychecks

Calculate each doctor's production at month's end and apply the corresponding percentages, then pay that amount by the 10th of the following month. For ROI compensation, divide the earned 12 percent of stock owned by 12 months and pay that amount on the second paycheck of the month.

This process means that owners who get compensation in both tiers get two paychecks every month. If appropriate, each partner will also receive a bonus check for the division of net profit at the end of the year. Pay any management compensation in either check. Dividing compensation this way benefits both doctor and practice, letting them budget effectively for the year.

Additional benefits

The Three-Tier Compensation Formula also facilitates buy-ins. Associates who decide to buy in receive production compensation, ROI, and a portion of net profit. The ROI income should help fund part of the buy-in.

The formula lets partners pursue their goals with appropriate compensation without adversely affecting the other owners. Partners cutting back on hours don't have to feel guilty. They receive less production and net profit compensation, yet still earn a fair ROI. Likewise, doctors who want extra income can do so without creating ill-will among their fellow partners.

It's critical that partners establish a fair compensation arrangement for themselves as well as associates. Even in the best formed partnerships, unequal workloads will affect the relationship. The Three-Tier Compensation Formula is a win-win for all concerned. Doctors receive appropriate compensation for the work they put into the practice, a fair return on their investment, and additional income as the practice continues to be profitable.

Chapter 20

Protect Yourself From Embezzlement

According to industry research, one out of 10 veterinary hospitals loses $10,000 or more each year from embezzlement. Although finding fault in a situation like this is never easy, veterinarians probably deserve the most blame. The veterinary profession is filled with trusting, caring individuals who never expect their staffs are capable of embezzlement. As a result, practice owners rarely use safeguards—and if they do, safeguards are rarely monitored.

As outrageous as it may seem, you must assume that at some point in your career you'll become a victim of embezzlement. And I'm not talking about a bottle of vitamins or shampoo, I'm talking $10,000 or more a year. To at least minimize losses, you must incorporate effective internal controls. The truth is, you can't really stop a determined embezzler, but you can make it hard on the thief. To help reduce the potential for embezzlement, consider instituting these standard business practices.

End-of-day procedures

Assuming your practice is computerized, I recommend you initiate this mandatory end-of-day procedure. If you haven't already done so, set the cash drawer at a base, say $100. Next, it's critical that you appoint two staff members as closers. Remember in kindergarten when you learned the buddy system—ensure safety by teaming with a buddy. The same holds true when keeping your practice safe. Multiple people involved in the end-of-day process means less chances of stealing. If your receptionist generates the end-of-day report and deposits funds in the bank, you've left the embezzlement door wide open. It's trite but true. Embezzlers are always the people you'd least suspect.

The closers print out the deposit report and compare it against the cash drawer. At the end of the day, the closers count out $100 and remove the remaining currency and checks. They then compare the cash, checks, and credit card transactions with the deposit report. All figures should balance. If not, the designated closers must find the error. If they can't, they should adjust the deposit, not the cash drawer. The drawer should always maintain its base amount to the exact penny.

Next, the closers must prepare the deposit form. Have them complete a daily deposit, even if you only go to the bank every other day. The closers should attach the bank receipt to the end-of-day report and place everything on the practice owner's desk. This creates a complete audit trail that shows all income was correctly entered into the computer and deposited into the bank. The owner initials the report and deposit receipt, then passes the bundle off to the bookkeeper.

End-of-day reports

All computer systems can generate several end-of-day reports. The two reports most important in protecting your practice are an itemized audit trail and a fee exception report. The itemized audit trail is a printout of all transactions, including voids, refunds, or credits issued to a client. Some programs even provide the initials of whoever made the transaction. The practice owner or manager should review the audit trail every day, paying particular attention to any negative transactions. This can help you pinpoint the most common form of embezzlement, which occurs with cash transactions.

Here's how it works. The receptionist invoices the client for $100. The client pays with cash, and the receptionist puts the $100 in the cash drawer. Later, that receptionist or another staff member who witnessed the transaction voids the invoice and pockets the cash. The end-of-day report will balance, and you're out $100. The only way you can detect a potential problem is with the itemized audit trail.

The fee exception report lists any charges that were more or less than the stated fee. Say you charge $20 for a given service, but the fee exception report shows transactions charged at $10 or $25. Again, this could indicate potential embezzlement. Either someone is giving 50 percent discounts or pocketing the extra $5.

Other safeguard tips

To take action today and protect yourself from future problems, consider implementing these policies in your practice.

Computer backups. It's in the best interest of you—and your practice—to back up your computer system each day. Also, you should make a weekly or monthly backup tape that's kept off site. This way, you won't lose vital information if your practice is damaged by fire, water, or other natural disasters. How often you decide to back up records depends on how much risk you're willing to take. I recommend you also make yearly backup tapes and store them in a safety-deposit box.

Password protection. This is by far one of the best ways to protect yourself from embezzlement or having your client list "borrowed" by a departing doctor. Although most computer systems offer this security option, few practices use it. Even when used, chances are the practice owner hasn't updated passwords in months or even years. I recommend using at least three levels of password protection: entry, manager, and owner. The entry level allows receptionists into areas necessary to invoice clients. The manager level can process voids, refunds, and other negative transactions. It also allows access to accounts receivable and inventory control. The owner level allows complete access.

Once you establish password protection, you must monitor and update it regularly. Most likely, the entry level will stay the same but the manager and owner levels should change every six months to a year, depending on turnover. You can also selectively protect any menu item, allowing you to be as open or secure as you please.

Check signing. The only person who should sign practice checks is the owner. Do not delegate this responsibility, even to a manager or bookkeeper. They can fill out checks, but the owner should sign them. There's no need to require all partners to sign checks. One owner's signature is sufficient. If you use signature stamps, I recommend you throw them out now. A signature stamp is an open invitation for embezzlers.

Bank statements. Request that all bank statements be sent directly to one of the owners' homes. That owner should immediately open the statement and review each transaction. Do this before passing it on to the bookkeeper or manager to reconcile.

Do you recognize your vendors' names? Many embezzlement scams involve a bogus company. The staff member issues a check to the fake company each month. You can deter this problem by having all bank statements sent directly to the practice owner's home for an initial review of vendor and signature.

Credit card transactions. Another prime embezzlement area is charge card processing. An employee can issue a credit to his or her account. Other times embezzlers may charge a cash invoice to a client's account, then pocket the money. An electronic terminal can reduce this problem. Also, I recommend you purchase a credit card printer for all charge card transactions. This not only speeds up processing, it lets you print an end-of-day daily transaction report similar to an itemized audit trail. Again, the owner or manager should review the transaction report and question any negative transactions.

Be alert and attentive. You are first a medical caregiver. But to succeed, you must also be a savvy business person. Establish effective safeguards to minimize embezzlement risks. Be aware of everything going on in your practice. If you even suspect theft, test your team. Mark a $20 bill, then ask a friend to buy a product with the cash and leave without requesting a receipt. Check the cash drawer soon afterward to see whether the marked bill is there. Periodically questioning transactions tells your staff that you are attentive to potential theft.

The information outlined here only scratches the surface of effective internal controls, but one point stands clear: Safeguarding any practice requires attention from the practice owner and manager. Don't get caught sleeping on the job.

Chapter 21

Develop a Hospital Business Team

I'm a firm believer in the team approach to management. Successful business owners surround themselves with professionals who possess skills in areas they lack. When faced with a challenging medical case, you probably wouldn't hesitate to seek a second opinion or refer the case to a specialist. So why not solicit assistance from other professionals when you have an apparent need?

It's a fact that veterinarians receive little, if any, practice-management training in veterinary school. Likewise, the average practice manager doesn't have the knowledge and skill of a certified public accountant, lawyer, or financial planner. Therefore, it's only smart that you have a savvy business team at your disposal.

Each practice has its own unique management needs. But, in general, your practice team should consist of a practice accountant, lawyer, management consultant, and financial planner.

Practice accountant: A valuable asset

Your practice accountant analyzes the financial information generated by your practice and helps you understand the figures on the report. He or she also reduces your tax liability while complying with state and federal laws and even assists with personal and practice financial planning.

An accountant should be more than a pencil pusher. Pencil pushers just write checks, complete payroll, compile financial records, and present monthly financial statements. They don't review this information or interpret it. In other words, pencil pushers are little more than glorified bookkeepers. So why waste an accountant's higher fees on bookkeeping work?

To ensure you receive the most benefit from your accountant, first decide which financial-related chores you'll do in-house and which you'll delegate to your accountant. Try to keep as much accounting and bookkeeping work in-house as possible. Today's technology offers programs to ease this workload, and besides, it makes no sense not to be computerized for your accounting needs. I suggest you use a stand-alone system for all accounting programs to limit the possibility of corruption. There are several excellent programs, such as One-Write Plus and Quick Books, that are inexpensive and user-friendly.

I also suggest you keep accounts payable in-house and—if you wish—produce your own monthly financial statements and budgets. Although you can complete payroll with these programs, it's better to hire a payroll company. These affordable companies prepare checks and send them to you signature-ready. They also prepare payroll and quarterly reports and W-2s at the end of the year.

Now that you've decided what tasks to keep in-house, review what your accountant should do. First, an accountant should interpret the financial information you provide. Just download your information onto a disk. You or your accountant shouldn't have to re-enter all the information. The accountant then works with the data, making adjustments as necessary before reviewing it with you.

Ideally, you should meet with your accountant quarterly or twice a year at minimum. One meeting should be at the end of the first quarter to evaluate the previous year's progress and set goals for the upcoming year. Conduct the second must-have meeting nine months into your fiscal year to prorate the year-end and make income projections. This is vital to making intelligent financial decisions about your practice. Quarterly meetings are best because your accountant can review changes in your financial position and compare them with last year's figures for the same quarter. The best accountants are familiar with the veterinary profession and can make comparisons to industry norms as well. This information is readily available through *Veterinary Economics* magazine if your accountant has the initiative to find it. Of course, veterinary-exclusive accountants will greatly benefit your practice because they understand the profession's unique circumstances and trends.

Whether you use a veterinary-specific accounting firm or a general CPA, your accountant should show interest in you as a person and in your business. Aside from the quarterly reviews, your accountant should ensure you pay only your fair share of taxes. He or she should stay current with tax codes and inform you of all deductions you're entitled to, such as Section 179, which lets you deduct up to $18,500—$19,000 on your 1999 taxes—in equipment purchases each year.

Your accountant should discuss options and offer advice regarding partnerships and incorporation, noting each option's advantages and disadvantages. Regarding financial planning, your accountant should discuss your future financial needs—your children's college education and your retirement—as well as building a new practice facility or buying a home.

As a consultant, I meet with clients' accountants whenever possible to discover each one's capabilities and evaluate the services provided. The sad truth is, eight out of 10 times I recommend the practice owner find a new accountant. Many accountants defend themselves by saying, "The veterinarian never asked me to do that." This excuse is unacceptable. Do you expect clients to be responsible for requesting vaccinations, heartworm, or other procedures when needed? Of course you don't. Just as it's your responsibility to inform clients what procedures their pets need to stay healthy, it's your accountant's responsibility to tell you how he or she can keep your practice healthy.

Practice lawyer: Your legal backbone
Without a doubt, there will be many occasions when you need a lawyer's expertise. Establishing a strong relationship with a lawyer will protect your interests.

I firmly believe no legal document should be signed without first having it reviewed by a qualified lawyer. If you're negotiating a lease with a landlord, drafting an employment contract, or writing a buy-sell agreement, you should involve a lawyer. It's wise to have the interested parties outline an agreement before meeting with the lawyer, so that he or she need only review the document and put it in legal form. This can also save substantial legal fees.

Consult a lawyer experienced in estate planning for wills and trust funds. This is an important area of financial planning that many people overlook. You can save—or lose—a great deal of money depending on how your estate is set up.

Aside from drafting legal documents and estate planning, you may also need your lawyer to help with personnel-management problems, personal-injury suits, or malpractice claims. If you don't already have a lawyer, find one who shares your business philosophy and begin forging a relationship today. When the need arises, you'll have someone you can turn to for assistance.

Management consultant: A professional beacon

Naturally, I'm somewhat prejudiced in this matter. But who better to tell you about the importance of a consultant to your business team than an actual consultant? A management consultant often sees things that you can't because you're too close to your practice. It becomes very personal to you, as it should.

This close attachment may mean you don't recognize those idiosyncrasies that aren't efficient or are even detrimental to your practice. Often things may have been done a certain way for so long that no one questions whether it's the most effective way. These problems can block future success. A consultant can examine your day-to-day operations with a trained, objective eye and propose ways to improve your practice and the services you provide.

Management consultants also can help with site analysis of a new or relocating practice, organize a new practice's initial management systems, and offer formal training programs for key staff members. A consultant can offer problem analysis and resolution, develop employee compensation plans, and assist in contract negotiations, partnership counseling, and key personnel employment counseling. Typically, many employees are more likely to listen to an outside "expert" than the practice owner.

It's an interesting fact that those businesses—whether a veterinary practice or any other business—that hire a consultant are usually in the top 20 percent of their industry. The irony is that those people who could benefit most from a consultant probably will never hire one because they don't see the value. But smart practice owners who want to become even better are likely the ones who will hire a consultant. If you decide to hire a consultant, choose one who specializes in the veterinary profession. First do your homework, talking to several consultants and requesting references, before making a decision.

Financial planner: Plotting your future

It's true that the more money you make, the more you spend. You may have had as much disposable income while in veterinary school as you have today. A financial planner can rectify this problem.

I'd like to share an all too real story, possibly the saddest story I've ever heard. A veterinarian who for 30 years devoted himself to his career now wants to retire—but he never put anything away for that retirement. While he worked long, hard hours to get ahead, his children grew up and his wife grew distant without him. Instead of reflecting on his years as a veterinarian with fondness, he resents the profession. This resentment has led to apathy, which has resulted in a deteriorating, outdated facility. He wants to sell the practice, but it's worth far less than the financial and emotional investment he's made. After 30 years, he's a bitter man.

The moral of the story: Now is the time to start planning for your future. A good financial planner will sit down with you and your spouse to discuss your current financial needs and devise a plan that will help ensure you have adequate funds for your children's college education or to enjoy retirement. I recommend you hire a fee-only financial planner. This approach means your financial adviser gets paid for working for you, not for selling any particular product or service, so there's no conflict of interest.

Your business team plays a key role in ensuring your business and personal success. A truly intelligent person knows his or her limitations and relies on people with complementary expertise. Isn't it time you formed your team today?

Chapter 22

Create a "10" Practice and Enjoy Life

When I speak at national and state conferences, I often ask attendees to rate their professional life on a scale of 1 to 10, with 10 meaning they're absolutely thrilled. People who rate their lives at 10 wake up every morning eager to get into work. At the day's end, they honestly believe they made a difference in a client's, pet's, or employee's life. They feel they're fairly compensated and truly enjoy what they do. On the other hand, people who rate their lives as 1s can't get out of bed in the morning and have to force themselves to come to work.

Out of the 700 people I asked this question to, how many do you think raised their hands when I asked, "Are you a 10?" Unfortunately, the answer is usually zero. Maybe one or two hands go up when I ask "9?" It's not until I hit 7, 6, and 5 that a lot of hands raise.

Why is this? I've worked with veterinarians most of my life and have yet to meet one who was forced to become a veterinarian. This is the life you chose, so why can't you rate it a 10?

When I'm asked to rate my professional life on a scale of 1 to 10, I answer with a resounding 15. I truly love my career. There is nothing else in this world I'd rather do. I eagerly anticipate each day, whether I spend it consulting at a veterinary hospital, lecturing at a state association, visiting veterinary students, or tinkering around my office. I wish all people could share this feeling of accomplishment and that everybody—whether a veterinarian, practice manager, technician, or receptionist—could rate their quality of professional life at 10 or higher.

A number of years ago, I learned something that had a significant impact on me. I was taught to ask myself, "What adds meaning and value to my life?" Once I found out, I learned to do more of those beneficial things and delegate other tasks to somebody else. Do employee performance reviews add meaning to your life? How about ordering inventory, then stocking it once it arrives? Does payroll get you jump-started each day?

If you're a practice owner and answered "no" to any of these questions, why are you doing them? Instead, delegate these tasks to your manager, bookkeeper, or associate. As practice owner, you have the right to choose how to spend your day. You can also choose whether your life rates a 10.

Personally, writing checks adds no value to my life. Why would I want to see my income depleted? Instead, I let my assistant do it. What tasks can you delegate to others?

I'm not advocating an anarchist mentality. You won't be able to do whatever you want whenever you want. Just be reasonable about how you spend your time. If you do more of the things you enjoy, it becomes easier to handle those tasks you don't.

Creating a "10" practice

What I consider a "10" practice may not resemble your idea, and that's the beauty of the concept: Each person has unique, individual criteria and perceptions as to what makes up a "10" practice. However, there are common factors that go into creating a "10" practice and others that we must overcome.

Consider when you first started out. You probably had a substantial debt load and a great deal of apprehension. The No. 1 factor that helped you become successful was fear of failure. Fear is a positive motivator and should be embraced. When fear no longer exists, we get complacent. Complacency leads to boredom, which leads to disinterest and eventually apathy. About this time, "clinical depression" sets in. You experience the "same ol', same ol'" every day. Once you recognize the importance of fear, you can change your practice environment before complacency sets in. Give your practice life an energy jolt by implementing new procedures, developing another profit center, renovating your facility, hiring an associate—anything to add a touch of fear.

Change is essential for success. If you don't enjoy any aspect of your practice, you must be willing to change it. It takes courage and guts, but harnessing fear will help you attain a "10" practice environment. There is a phenomenon called "life sickness." Much like seasickness, life sickness is caused by an unwillingness to change your position even though everything else around you is rocking and rolling. You can become life sick if you don't accept the fact that change is necessary and important—the essence of success. This is your opportunity to make a difference.

Create your practice vision

Vision is having an acute sense of the possible. I believe every single practice owner should develop a vision statement for his or her practice. Vision statements explain the practice's direction to the staff. The people who provide this direction are the practice owners.

Dr. Ed Epperson created the following vision statement for his eight-doctor small animal practice—it's one of the best I've ever read. It truly provides a sense of what this practice is all about:

A "10" Practice:

I am in the process of creating a "10" practice. That project will be finished when I cease to practice. The most important factor in my relationship is the word "I." What is an "I" (me)? I see myself as a visionary, healer and humorist. Therefore my job is to create a vision, heal, and have fun.

VISIONARY—I will create the model health care context that will empower veterinarians during the next 100 years. I was a thing manipulating other things (clients); who I am now is SERVICE. I am contribution. I speak and listen from that way of being. From that base, I recommend dentistry and other services—not as a survival speech to pay the rent but as a pure, unadulterated contribution. I speak, "How may I assist you?" and "What project shall we work on?" through a conversation for action.

Each person on my staff will be empowered to speak and listen as if they were me. They can make promises for me and expect me to keep them. There will be an unconditional commitment to excellence, taking care of people, profitability, economic freedom, and having fun. I promise each employee that they will never have to work with an "8" or lower. I promise that a "9" will have 30 days or less to become a "10." Each employee must agree to be supported by each of the others to constantly be a "10."

I am unconditionally committed to being a standard for our clients having healthy pets. We will educate, treat and protect against disease and behavioral problems in such a way that having a pet is maximally rewarding and never a burden. I see the pet being so healthy that the human chooses to mimic the way that created that result.

Our gross practice income will be $500,000 or more. That's $2,000 a day for 250 days. We will earn $166 an hour while the hospital is open and $250 a doctor an hour, which equals $2,000 divided by eight. This goal is simply a measurement of the public's excitement and acceptance of our new service. We love ourselves and deserve the best of everything.

P.S. We will collect 98 percent of the money charged.

HEALER—It's important that I avoid identifying myself as the employer, tax payer, custodian, public relations person, etc. Who I am and what I am is a healer, missionary, and humorist. I am educated and intuitive. I will use my skills expertly to produce miraculous results in health care. I promise to stay current and also to refer all cases that I cannot handle excellently.

LOCALITY—A "10" facility has beauty (colors, pictures), music (enlivening). We will use tapes that serve our purpose. It will be clean and smell good, and laughter will be very common.

PROFITABILITY—We can't be too profitable. Our fee structure combined with our volume will allow us to provide:
1) The best in radiographs, lab tests, surgery, and medicine.
2) The best salaries for our "10" employees.
3) Bonuses based on profitability.

4) Our fees will force us to be great. We must participate like people expensive and worth it.

FUN—I demand that any employee call me to task if I am not having fun. They need to know that counseling a client on how to handle their grief over losing a pet is enjoyable and not a laughing matter. I have fun crying. So, I promise to have fun every minute of every day for the rest of my life.

This is one doctor's vision of his "10" practice. In reading this vision statement, you get a clear picture of his goals. It's critical that the owner tell everyone on staff exactly what he or she wants to accomplish. Without leadership at the top, no business will ever succeed.

Develop and state a constitution for your practice

Today, I want you unconditionally to commit to excellence in every thing you do. Commit to getting things done today because we don't have time tomorrow.

Enjoy every single minute of the day. This helps your staff to center on specific goals and targets. State your vision to yourself as well as your staff and live that vision.

The staff also must commit to your vision, and you can't adjust the vision to fit your staff. It's OK if an employee can't commit. That person just can't be on your staff.

Tell employees that if you find another person better than them, you will hire that person and replace them. This isn't a threat. It's a promise that you will have a team of "10s" who are committed to the practice's vision of excellence.

Once you announce excellence, you have to be excellent. The ripple effect of deciding to offer excellence is staggering. It's impossible to do enough for another person. The more you give, the more you get. The world is starving for excellence. Finding a business that's committed to excellence is difficult. Once people do, they stick with it. To become a "10" practice, you must:
- Be willing to overcome fear.
- Create and maintain a vision.

- Develop a "10" staff without compromise.
- Commit to excellence.
- Have a "10" facility.
- Serve clients who want excellence.
- Pay the highest salaries and bonuses.

A "10" practice will afford you high-quality professional and personal lives, economic rewards, and the achievement of excellence. The one absolute key for success is to not only meet clients' expectations but exceed them. What can you do to accomplish this? Recognize clients and their pets by name as they enter the practice. Use an exam-room report card to document the comprehensive physical exam. Call clients after discharging their pets to inquire about their progress. And the list goes on and on.

The veterinary profession is highly revered. Veterinarian is almost always among the top three responses when you ask children, "What do you want to be when you grow up?"

I've devoted my life to veterinary practice management. Above all else, I wish to make a difference in this world, both personally and professionally. Personally, I wish to be a good person, a wonderful husband, and raise three children who will also have a positive impact on this world. Professionally, I would like to teach veterinarians how to practice smarter, not harder. I want people to view this profession as a paragon of customer service. I'm sure you often hear, "I wish my doctor cared for me as well as you care for my pet." I want that comment stated not only daily but hourly.

You can set the standard for others to follow. I'll end this book with the same statement I end my seminars with because I know by the session's end people realize how valuable this statement is:

Love your clients so much, care for them and their pets so well that they do not want to leave your practice for fear of a harsher world outside your doors. Make a difference in this world and in this profession. We only have a short time to do so. Today is the beginning of the rest of your life!

Figures List

Support Materials List

Avian Report Card

For:

_____

OWNER

_____

PET'S NAME

_____/_____/_____

DATE

---

1. General Appearance
- ❑ Normal
- ❑ Fluffed
- ❑ Other _____

2. General Attitude
- ❑ Normal
- ❑ Increased Activity
- ❑ Decreased Activity

3. Eyes
- ❑ Normal
- ❑ Abscess
- ❑ Ulceration
- ❑ Other _____

4. Feathering
- ❑ Normal
- ❑ Missing Feathers
- ❑ Cysts
- ❑ Other _____

5. Choanal Slit
- ❑ Normal
- ❑ Redness
- ❑ Blunted Papilla
- ❑ Plaques
- ❑ Other _____

6. Cloaca
- ❑ Normal
- ❑ Growths
- ❑ Other _____

7. Abdomen
- ❑ Normal
- ❑ Masses
- ❑ Other _____

8. Character of Droppings
- ❑ Normal
- ❑ Increased Urates
- ❑ Increased Solids
- ❑ Other _____

❑ **Diagnosis / Description**

(Numbers below correspond to numbers above)

_____

_____

_____

_____

_____

_____

_____

_____

DR. _____

Recommendations

_____

_____

_____

_____

_____

_____

_____

_____

Need _____ **in** ____ **days**

EQUINE REPORT CARD

V-C-M INC

For:

OWNER _____

HORSE _____

DATE ____/____/____

Vaccination Program

☐ Up to Date
☐ Vac. Due: Tetanus _____ EEE/WEE _____ Flu _____ Rhino _____ PHF _____ Strangles _____
☐ Vac. Given: Tetanus _____ EEE/WEE _____ Flu _____ Rhino _____ PHF _____ Strangles _____

1. Coat & Skin

☐ Appears normal ☐ Oily ☐ Itchy
☐ Dull ☐ Shedding ☐ Parasites
☐ Scaly ☐ Matted ☐ Other: _____
☐ Dry ☐ Tumors

2. Eyes

☐ Appear normal ☐ Infection: L___ R___
☐ Discharge: L___ R___ ☐ Cataract: L___ R___
☐ Inflamed: L___ R___ ☐ Other
☐ Eyelid Deformities

3. Ears

☐ Appears normal ☐ Tumor: L___ R___
☐ Inflamed ☐ Excessive Hair
☐ Itchy ☐ Other _____
☐ Mites

4. Nose & Throat

☐ Appears normal ☐ Enlarged Lymph Glands
☐ Nasal Discharge ☐ Other _____
☐ Inflamed Throat

5. Mouth, Teeth, Gums

☐ Appears normal ☐ Inflamed Lips
☐ Broken Teeth ☐ Loose Teeth
☐ Sharp Edges ☐ Pyorrhea
☐ Ulcers ☐ Other _____
☐ Tumors

6. Legs & Hooves

☐ Appears normal ☐ Joint Problems
☐ Lameness ☐ Hoof Problems
☐ Damaged Ligaments ☐ Other _____

7. Heart

☐ Appears normal ☐ Fast
☐ Murmur ☐ Other _____
☐ Slow

8. Abdomen

☐ Appears normal ☐ Abnormal Mass
☐ Enlarged Organs ☐ Painful
☐ Fluid ☐ Other _____

9. Lungs

☐ Appears normal ☐ Breathing Difficulty
☐ Abnormal sound ☐ Rapid Respiration
☐ Coughing ☐ Other _____
☐ Congestion

10. Gastrointestinal System

☐ Appears normal ☐ Abnormal Feces
☐ Palpation - OK ☐ Parasites
☐ Colic History ☐ Anorexia
☐ Sounds: L___ R___

11. Urogenital System

☐ Abnormal urination ☐ Mammary tumors
☐ Discharge ☐ Other _____
☐ Abnormal testicles

12. Central Nervous System

☐ Appears Normal ☐ Depression
☐ Seizures ☐ Behavior Problems

13. Diet

☐ Excellent ☐ Vitamins needed
☐ Good ☐ Improvement necessary

Coggins Test
☐ Negative
☐ Positive
☐ Recommended

Fecal Test
☐ Negative
☐ Positive
☐ Recommended

☐ **Diagnosis / Description**
(Numbers below correspond to numbers above)

_____
_____
_____
_____
_____
_____
_____
_____
_____
_____
_____

Recommendations

_____
_____
_____
_____
_____
_____
_____
_____
_____
_____

DR. _____

Need _____ in _____ days

- JOB DESCRIPTION -

HOSPITAL ADMINISTRATOR

Reports To:
Board Of Directors

Function:
Responsible for all accounting and financial control functions, including financial planning, budgeting, control and reporting systems, and financial analyses. Through financial counsel and the application of financial tools, ensures that hospital management has adequate visibility of operations.

Experience Requirements:
The position requires demonstrated competence in the theory and practice of accounting and financial control. The successful candidate must have expertise in budgeting, financial reporting, and financial analysis. A qualified candidate should have had working exposure to all aspects of a business enterprise. Successful supervisory experience is mandatory. Hospital or veterinary experience would be helpful, but is not required.

Education Requirements:
College degree is required.

Personal Requirements:
The successful candidate must be intelligent, self-confident, and energetic. He must possess obvious leadership qualities and supervisory abilities. He must be sufficiently adaptable to operate effectively in different roles with a variety of people within and outside the hospital.

The qualified candidate must possess a high degree of general business acumen. He must also be attuned to the variables which make for successful financial management. He must be creative, yet able to develop and implement practical programs. He must possess good judgment and the willingness and capability for making decisions. He must be interested in contributing substantively to successful hospital performance and growth.

Duties and Responsibilities:

1. Recommends policies governing financial control and accounting practices.

2. Provides counsel to hospital management on all accounting and financial matters.

3. Assists in establishing and maintaining sound financial control and reporting

systems covering all operations; exercises necessary functional authority to ensure that control policies and procedures are followed.

4. Assists in conducting long-range financial planning.

5. Develops operating budgets.

6. Assists in analyzing and interpreting financial data for management with emphasis on identifying problems, identifying trends, and forecasting the financial consequences of alternative decisions.

7. Ensures that appropriate accounting records are maintained on all assets, liabilities, and transactions.

8. Ensures the timely preparation of financial statements.

9. Assists in developing and maintaining appropriate cash flow projections and controls; continually reviews the hospital's cash position to ensure that adequate funds are available to meet outstanding and planned commitments.

10. Maintains an appropriate chart of accounts.

11. Develops and maintains suitable procedures for controlling and valuing inventories.

12. Develops and maintains suitable procedures for handling cash and all other assets to protect the hospital from loss through negligence or dishonesty.

13. Participates in the analysis of financing requirements; develops and recommends appropriate methods of financing.

14. Acts as liaison with banks, arranging financing when required.

15. Administers all insurance activities, including recommendations regarding the determination of risk and the placement of coverage.

16. Ensures that accounting practices are in accordance with the requirements of regulatory bodies and that reports required by such organizations are prepared and submitted.

17. Acts as immediate contact with the hospital's independent auditors.

18. Assists in the investigation, analysis, and appraisal of hospital expansion activities.

19. Performs special analytical, statistical, and financial studies as required.

20. Prepares appropriate forms and reports relative to payroll, property, and sales tax compliance.

21. Assists in contract negotiations, ensuring that agreements are sound from a financial standpoint.

22. Through leadership, supervision, and management control, maintains a work group which effectively executes its assigned functions, and which is highly responsive to management needs for control, information, and analysis.

23. Maintains knowledge of current developments in accounting theory and practice, and in financial techniques for measurement, analysis, and planning.

24. Acts as liaison with hospital attorney to access and inform on legal ramifications of contracts, agreements, etc. Will recommend or advise on policies where appropriate.

25. Assists in interviewing applicants for supervisory positions.

26. Assists in developing and maintaining salary schedules and job evaluations for all employees.

- JOB DESCRIPTION -

RECEPTIONIST / CASHIER

Job Summary:
Under direction of the hospital's practice manager, conducts a variety of clerical functions relevant to the operation of a small animal hospital, including establishing satisfactory credit arrangements in accordance with hospital policies and procedures.

Minimum Qualifications:

Knowledge Of: General office practices and procedures including filing systems; receptionist and telephone techniques

Ability To: Perform clerical work with speed and accuracy;
Use a ten key adding machine and multiple line telephone;
Typing speed of at least 45 words per minute;
Greet client clients graciously and recognize the responsibilities involved in responding to client questions;
Keep simple records;
Understand and carry out oral and written directions;
Proficiently handle all forms of monies;
Maintain a neat professional appearance;
Maintain a harmonious and cooperative relationship with those contacted in the course of work

Education: Equivalent to completion of 12th grade

Experience: At least two years recent experience in general office work with increasing responsibilities

Recent experience at a veterinary hospital is preferred.

Specific Duties:

1. Receives all incoming phone calls.

2. Schedules all appointments.

3. Receives clients as they arrive and establishes the purpose of each visit.

4. Updates the existing medical file and history card or collects sufficient information to prepare a new file.

5. Escorts clients from the waiting room to the examination area.

6. Receives payments for services rendered.

7. Establishes credit in accordance with hospital policies and procedures and assures that the posting clerk has adequate information to credit accounts correctly.

8. Reviews past due accounts and attempts to personally contact the individuals concerned; decides which accounts will be turned over to the credit bureau and

which will later be subjected to direct collection.

9. Answers questions regarding the status of hospitalized animals as directed by the attending veterinarian.

10. Prepares vaccine reminder cards.

11. Maintains the appearance of the business office.

12. Maintains an accurate inventory of office supplies and over-the-counter medications.

13. Refiles medical records and files medical reports into the appropriate medical records.

14. Refills prescriptions in accordance with hospital policies and procedures.

15. Prepares the daily posting report; balances cash and checks daily; makes daily bank deposit.

16. Occasionally types letters.

17. Other related duties as assigned.

- Job Description -

RECEPTIONIST

INTRODUCTION

The purpose of this position is to serve as receptionist at the ABC Veterinary Hospital, to perform record keeping duties, to perform clerical duties related to animal patient care and treatment, and to provide miscellaneous support to the Veterinary Practice Manager and the staff. This position requires a practical knowledge of hospital organization and services, the basic rules and regulations governing visitors and animal patient treatment, data transcribing, word processing, and a practical knowledge of the standard procedures, veterinary records, and terminology used in the hospital.

MAJOR GOALS

- To be efficient, very pleasant, courteous, polite, concerned, and helpful to all clients under all conditions and at all times.
- To see that the client leaves the office with another visit scheduled for their continued pet health care. Specifically, schedule a follow-up, recheck, or re-vaccination appointment or set up a reminder for future health care needs.
- To keep the office organized, ensuring a smooth and efficient client flow.
- To see that appointments remain on schedule by being totally familiar with times required for different procedures and problems, scheduling accordingly.

MAJOR DUTIES

- Follow Employee General Policies.
- Put client/pet records that are to be seen that day in alphabetical order. Records are obtained from the computer by using option 221.
- Answer the telephone with a smile.
- Greet clients with a smile and try to address both client and pet by name.
- Determine the client flow, i.e., the order to the exam room, which doctor sees the client, etc.
- Coordinate client and pet flow.
  - Usher clients into exam room.
  - Be sure the exam room has been properly cleaned and deodorized. If not, do so immediately and/or use another room.
  - Complete the client admission form.
  - Be sure all routine procedures such as vaccinations, heartworm tests, etc. are up-to-date.
  - Take pet record from reception area and place in appropriate exam room door holder.
  - Admit pets for boarding, grooming, surgery, etc. and take them to ward.
    - Put pet belongings in appropriate place.
    - Write up cage card.
    - Place record in appropriately colored folder.
  - Call for pets being released and be sure all pets being released are clean and presentable.
  - Be sure personal property is returned to the client.
  - Counsel clients regarding nutrition, behavioral problems, obesity, worm problems, geriatric care, flea problems, pre- and post-operative care, treatment

instructions, etc.
- Provide clients with appropriate handout literature for the pet's medical condition, problem, nutrition, etc. All clients should leave with some sort of literature.
- Promote sales of our products.
- Ask all clients: "Do you have enough (flea supplies/shampoo/vitamins/etc.) to last until your next visit?"
- Client departure.
  - See that all clients have a reappointment for their continued pet health care.
  - All clients are asked if they have any questions or problems. Resolve all questions and problems.
  - Use common sense, e.g., euthanasia, cancer, severe injury—don't ask, "Did everything go okay?"
- Collecting After Visit
  - Verify that all items on the fee sheet are entered into the computer invoice.
  - First, ask client if everything was okay or if they have any questions.
  - Itemize charges as much as possible.
  - If minor grumbling over charges - handle yourself. An example of an acceptable response might be, "Pets get the same good care, lab work, and medication as people...Good medicine isn't inexpensive..."
  - If major grumbling or you can't handle, call the doctor involved.
  - If unhappy with services/treatment, ascertain the problem and handle. If unable to do so, call the doctor involved.
  - Never let a client leave the clinic without handling all negative situations.
  - Process client payments - I.e., cash drawer and computer.
  - Review discharge information or handouts with client.
- Making appointments
  - Responsible for scheduling all appointments.
  - Try to make appointments as early in the day as possible.
  - Try to make appointments during weekdays. Saturday fills up quickly.
  - Concentrate on filling the current day with appointments.
  - Clients that are no-shows are called within five minutes to see if they are on their way. If not, then reschedule an appointment and enter "no show - call and remind" after their name.
  - If unable to reach the client that is a no-show, enter their name in the message book and continue calling until they are contacted.
  - Be sure appointments are made with the correct DVM.
  - Be sure release appointments, if necessary, are made when the animal is dropped off.
  - Be sure reappointments are made. If the reappointment is more than five weeks in the future, "We'll call and remind you" and mark as such in the appointment book.
  - If vaccination, intestinal problem, or general illness, remind the client toward the end of the conversation to bring in a bowel movement sample (in plastic wrap, butter cup, etc.) and, if 6 years old or older, a urine sample. "Give it to us as soon as you come in, so we can start the test early."
  - Tell the client that their pet "needs" or "is now overdue" or "it is very important." Convince the client to make the appointment. The client needs our services in order to keep their pet healthy and avoid future costs.
  - Offer only two times on a particular date you have selected to choose from for their appointment.
  - If surgery is planned, remind client no food after midnight; water is okay till 7:00 a.m.

- Medication and records
  - If from another doctor, or medication involved, remind the client to bring any records or medication the pet is on.
- Bathing/Grooming
  - Ask all clients if they want a medicated and/or flea bath, and/or dip. Get complete instructions on how they want the animal groomed. Check for extensive matting and get accurate quote from groomer or office manager.
- Boarding
  - Ask all clients if they want a bath, nail trim, etc. done while boarding.
  - Ask all clients if they would like a check-up, worm test, etc. while boarding.
  - Make sure vaccines are up to date or that proof of such is brought with pet.
- Miscellaneous
  - If growth or tumor removal, have client point out location to you and mark with a felt marker.
  - Be sure all necessary release statements are signed.
  - Be sure no client waits any longer than 10 minutes before being put in an exam room.
  - Hand out client surveys, quizzes, suckers, coloring books, etc.
  - Monitor reception room cleanliness and clean if necessary.
  - Help with cleaning the entire area between hours.

- JOB DESCRIPTION -

EXAM-ROOM TECHNICIAN

INTRODUCTION

The purpose of this position is to assist with treatments, computerize all transactions, maintain inventory, monitor hospitalized pets, run routine in-house lab work, and client education. This is an overview of the position and is not limited to the major duties.

MAJOR DUTIES

- Assist in exam rooms by getting weight, temperature and brief history. Restrain animals during exam. Computerize highlighted Patient Visit Forms and prepare any needed prescriptions. Do routine suture removals, nail trims and weight checks.
- Basic client education, including puppy/kitten care, heartworms and nutrition.
- Assist with morning rotations of animals in kennel. Make sure all animals get needed medication. Treat routine surgical patients from previous day.
- Maintain any treatments requested by doctor. Mark all services rendered on tracking form.
- Have supplies prepared for exams and appointments.
- Run fecals, heartworm tests, urinalysis and FeLV tests as needed. Keep area clean.
- Monitor lab supplies and have all forms and tubes labeled for any scheduled blood work. After blood has been drawn, spin down and wrap up in form. Take lab results over the phone. Order lab supplies, as needed.
- Monitor pets in clinic to be sure they are comfortable and clean. Clean cages as needed. Oversee kennel duties.
- Order prescription pet foods on Mondays and Thursdays.
- Enter fees into the computer for:
    - Surgery/hospitalized patients, using in-house tracking forms. Call pets' owners to advise of pets' statuses.
    - Boarding pets: Take files and anything left with pet, forward on the day going home.
- Perform and assist in dental procedures.
- Assist in taking, developing and maintaining x-rays as needed.
- Maintain animal records by recording all conversations with clients and any work done. Work closely with doctors and follow-up on additional work needed.
- Prepare any prescriptions that need to be dispensed.
- Admit and release boarders.
- Start computer in morning, when needed.
- Inventory Control
    - Maintain adequate supplies.
    - Order, when necessary.
    - Negotiate best prices.
    - Unpack boxes and check-off packing lists.
    - Stock and store.
    - Maintain inventory in computer.
- Help keep hospital clean and orderly.
- Perform any other duties requested by the doctor or practice manager.

- JOB DESCRIPTION -

VETERINARY TECHNICIAN

INTRODUCTION

The Veterinary Technician/Assistant is responsible for beginning the procedures for examination once the receptionist has weighed the pet and placed it and the owner in the exam room. Restraint of the pet during exam and treatment may be necessary. Ensuring medications are ready and explaining their use will be necessary. Answer any extraneous questions the client may have, give pertinent literature and guide the client out to receptionist for payment processing.

PURPOSE

- To be efficient, very pleasant, courteous, polite, concerned and helpful to all clients under all conditions and at all times.
- To see that the client leaves the office with another visit scheduled for their continued pet health care. Contribute your part to the three "R's": recall, reminder, rescheduled recheck appointment.
- To keep the office organized, ensuring a smooth and efficient client flow.
- To recommend all necessary laboratory work, such as pre-anesthetic profiles, heartworm tests, feline leukemia tests, geriatric physicals, that are necessary for optimum patient care.
- To recommend all vaccinations that are necessary for optimum patient care.
- To recommend products such as flea control, vitamins, diets and dentals that are necessary for optimum patient care.
- To counsel clients regarding behavioral problems, obesity, geriatric care, nutritional problems, flea control, etc.

SPECIFIC DUTIES

- Follow ABC Hospital general policies.
- Greet client with and smile. Address both the client and patient by name.
- Assist in getting animal on exam room table and obtain temperature.
- Get additional information on animal's reason for presentation to the clinic.
- Set up fecal, urine for examination.
- Call doctor to exam room.
- Aid in restraining animal for examination and treatment by doctor.
- Get results of lab work ready for doctor.
- Anticipate vaccines or other medications doctor will need to treat animal and have ready.
- Anticipate medications that need to be sent home with pet and count pills and prepare labels.
- Get any literature ready that is pertinent to the pet's problem and owner's questions.
- Have Exam Room Report Card prepared for doctor to fill out.
- Show client how to give medications to pet.
- Answer any additional questions and escort client to reception area for payment processing.
- Check exam room drawers and remove used syringes and other materials. Clean table. Sweep and spot clean floor, if necessary.
- Keep lab and pharmacy area neat and free of dirty items.

ADDITIONAL INFORMATION AND METHODS

- The exam room technician should attempt to market the services of the practice, as well as inform the client about any preventative procedures necessary to their pet's health.
  - Recommend vaccinations.
  - Recommend laboratory procedures, such as pre-anesthetic profiles, fecals, urinalysis, heartworm check, FeLV testing, etc.
  - Correction of abnormalities found, such as skin problems, fleas, etc.
- Sample scripts:
  - "I certainly wouldn't want to be anesthetized without first being checked out thoroughly to be sure it would be safe."
  - "It's been six months. We should check Clyde for worms."
  - "Missy is over 6 years old. We should do a urinanalysis. Kidney disease is the most common cause of death in middle age and older pets."
  - "We should give Fido a medicated flea bath to make him more comfortable and send him home nice and clean."
  - "While Sheba is under anesthetic for neutering, it would be a good time to clean her teeth and/or remove that growth."
  - "This would be a good opportunity to get those long toe nails taken care of."
- At departure of client:
  - Ensure that all reminders and recalls have been generated. Make sure the receptionist knows when the doctor wants the animal seen again for follow-up recheck exam and that an appointment is set.
  - All clients are asked if they have any questions or problems. Resolve all questions and problems.
  - Consider handing out your business card. "Here is my card. If you have any questions or problems, feel free to call."

- JOB DESCRIPTION -

VETERINARY TECHNICIAN/ASSISTANT

INTRODUCTION

The Veterinary Technician/Assistant is responsible for beginning the procedures for examination. First, the animal is weighed and the weight recorded on the client card, the temperature is taken and recorded and medical history is taken on an existing client.

It may be necessary for the Vet Tech to help restrain the pet during the examination and treatment. If injections are needed, the Vet Tech will give those.

OTHER DUTIES

- Setting up and reading fecals under the microscope and looking for parasites; reading blood work under microscope looking for heartworms.

- Dispensing medication which the doctor has prescribed.

- Taking drug inventory and keeping supplies for cleaning, animal food, paper towels, etc. current.

- Prepping an animal for surgery.

- Assisting in surgery.

- Assisting with the operation of the anesthesia machine.

- Preparing surgery packs and cutting surgery drapes.

- Cleaning and autoclaving syringes and needles.

- Assisting with x-rays.

- Supervising kennel help and being responsible for the cleanliness of the hospital—upstairs and downstairs.

- It is imperative that the wards and kennels be kept clean and disinfected.

- Thoroughly cleaning autoclave every month.

- Assisting with the dog walking, cage cleaning and general hospital cleaning.

- Checking on every animal in hospital and reporting to doctor.

- After the client leaves the exam room, the table should be cleaned and the room made ready for the next client.

- Be sure supplies are always available in exam rooms and treatment room.

- See that necessary literature is always available for you or doctor to give to client.

- Throughout the day, check on in-patients and report any abnormalities to doctor.

- The Vet Tech is responsible for dental cleanings.

- Keeping the treatment area clean and free of dirty items used during treatment.

171

- JOB DESCRIPTION -

SURGICAL ASSISTANT

INTRODUCTION

The purpose of this position is to prepare, assist and monitor all surgical patients and procedures. This is an overview of the position and is not limited to the duties listed.

MAJOR DUTIES

- Assist with morning kennel procedures by rotating, feeding and cleaning animals.
- Review surgery schedule and set up surgeries going home that day first.
- Get together all necessary instruments and equipment needed.
- Prepare anesthetic according to pet's weight and needs. Have anesthetic machine and trach tube ready, if needed.
- Assist doctor with surgical procedures.
- Clean up animals following surgery, give injection of antibiotics and trim nails. Check file to see if anything else is needed while pet is in the hospital.
- Monitor pet throughout recovery.
- Prepare for next surgery until all are completed.
- Clean and sterilize all instruments, gloves, drapes and equipment used, so that it will be ready the next time they are needed.
- Keep log of all surgeries done.
- Post all charges to tracking form.
- Assist in taking and developing x-rays, when needed.
- Assist doctors or other staff, when needed.
- Review sterilization dates on bone instruments and re-sterilize as needed.
- Maintain all anesthetic machines, autoclave, and any other equipment used in surgery.
- Maintain inventory on all suture or surgery supplies and place on want list, if needed.
- Thoroughly clean surgery room daily and work area weekly.
- Perform any other duties that are requested by the doctor or practice manager.

- JOB DESCRIPTION -

WARD ATTENDANT

Job Summary:

Under direction of the Nursing Supervisor, provides for the constant cleanliness of cages, runs and ward areas and the proper feeding and care of all hospitalized animals.

Specific Duties:

1. Cleans and sanitizes all cages, runs, wards and related areas;

2. Gives baths (ordinary cleansing, flea, medicated) and does whatever grooming as may be necessary to the treatment and constant cleanliness of each animal;

3. Recognizes and records any unusual condition or abnormal behavior of any hospitalized animal; observes animals recovering from anesthesia;

4. Feeds each animal as prescribed by the attending D.V.M. and records appetites; keeps kitchen area clean and neat;

5. Receives animals to be admitted for hospital care and is responsible for their proper identification and for recording their respective locations;

6. Releases animals to their owners as directed by the attending doctor and office manager and insures that every animal released is clean and properly groomed;

7. Assists doctors, nurses, treatment assistants and other personnel with the administration of medications or with restraint;

8. Other duties assigned as required;

Minimum Qualifications:

Knowledge Of: Cleaning and disinfecting methods and the use and care of cleaning materials and equipment;

Proper methods of animal restraint;

Ability To: Use cleaning materials and equipment with skill and efficiency;

Perform moderately heavy physical labor;

Sympathetically and patiently treat sick and injured animals;

Learn to administer medications and recognize abnormal conditions;

Understand and carry out oral and written directions;

Maintain cooperative relationships with those contacted in the course of work;

Education: Equivalent to completion of 12th grade

Desirable Qualifications:

Knowledge of: Basic pharmacology; supplemental courses in the field of Biological Science, Anatomy, and Physiology, Nursing, Medical Assisting or Veterinary Technology;

Experience: Previous experience in a veterinary hospital or related medical field.

- JOB DESCRIPTION -

DELIVERY AND DRUG ROOM CLERK

Job Summary:

Under direction of the Nursing Supervisor and Drug Purchasing Agent, operates a light truck in furnishing a pick-up and delivery service for the clinics as required; assumes responsibility for truck maintenance and cleanliness; has charge of the drug room in receiving, storing, issuing and delivering drug supplies; keeps accurate inventory of all supplies; other duties as assigned and required.

Specific Duties:

1. Furnishes clinics with require medical supplies; transports animals between clinics whenever required; brings blood and urine samples to the central hospital for processing;
2. Transports dead animals to the crematorium;
3. Delivers bank deposits, postage meters, mail and performs any errand duties deemed necessary;
4. Keeps truck maintained with gas and oil, checks tires and battery, washes truck and cleans interior; arranges for vehicle maintenance;
5. Keeps drug room clean and neat; receives shipments as they arrive and is responsible for their proper storage; keeps accurate inventory of all drug supplies issued and received;
6. Assists purchasing agent in selecting, locating and/or receiving new shipments;
7. Other duties may include general hospital maintenance, assisting doctors, nurses or kennel help;

Minimum Qualifications:

License:	Possession of a valid state Operator's License.
Knowledge of:	Safe driving practices and principles of vehicle preventative maintenance;
Ability to:	Drive a light truck safely and efficiently;
	Lift, load and unload heavy boxes, animals, etc.;
	Keep simple records;
	Understand and carry out oral and written directions;
	Maintain cooperative relationships with those contacted in the course of work;
Education:	Equivalent to completion of 12th grade

Desirable Qualifications:

Knowledge of:	Rules and procedures regulating freight and parcel shipments; Stock inventory procedures; Basic pharmacology
Experience:	Recent work experience involving vehicle driving

- JOB DESCRIPTION -

HOSPITAL MAINTENANCE PERSON

INTRODUCTION

The purpose of this position is to provide upkeep and repairs to the grounds and building of the ABC Veterinary Hospital. Duties will include:

- All aspects of lawn, landscaping and driveway care.
- Maintenance of all buildings, indoor and outdoor.
- Maintenance of all equipment and tools used in job assignments.
- Maintenance of practice and farm vehicles.
- Maintenance of equine hospital facilities and stable area.

MAJOR DUTIES

The following duties will be performed by the Hospital Maintenance Person. Detailed instructions can be found in the work manual.

- The primary, overriding duty is to keep the appearance of the hospital immaculate. Our clientele judge our hospital by what they can easily see.
- Mowing, cleaning, painting, leaf and snow removal, driveway maintenance, fence maintenance, landscaping, garbage removal.
- Maintaining equipment used to complete job assignments and keeping such equipment and tools in good working condition. Doing minor repairs on such equipment as needed and notifying management as to major repairs needed or new equipment necessary to adequately complete assignments. Also, keeping equipment and tools put away in proper storage areas.
- Care of practice and farm vehicles including inside and outside cleaning, checking and replenishing fluids, checking tire pressure, and notifying management when tune-ups or repairs beyond maintenance person's expertise are needed.
- Minor repair work inside hospitals including, but not limited to, lighting, painting, minor electrical, plumbing, and carpentry work, and maintenance of workshop and tools.
- Care of equine patients including stall cleaning, feeding, watering and cleaning of barn and equine clinic interiors. Sometimes helping medical staff with handling equine patients.
- At the request of staff, helping in the hospital proper with cleaning or restraining animals or other chores that may need doing.

CONTROLS OVER WORK

Work assignments will be completed in accordance with operating instructions. Works under loose supervision of office manager and veterinary practice manager who indicates general assignments, limitations, and priorities. The majority of the work involves recurring assignments that are performed independently. Personal use of judgement in selecting methods, establishing priorities and completing jobs is strongly encouraged. Work is reviewed in terms of adequacy of the services performed, compliance with operating instructions and the amount of supervision and verbal instruction necessary.

OTHER SIGNIFICANT FACTS

Apply knowledge and skills in building and grounds maintenance. Some knowledge of electrical, plumbing and carpentry work. Some knowledge of automotive maintenance. Knowledge of small machine maintenance.

Physical effort: Work may require lifting and carrying weight upwards of 100 lbs. Climbing ladders, running lawn equipment and farm equipment (tractor, manure spreader and hay baler), snow plowing, shoveling snow and manure.
Working conditions: Larger percentage of work will be outdoors with indoor work required as well. Outdoor work in winter time will be necessary. Exposure to animal wastes and animal medical wastes may occur.

BATHER / KENNEL ASSISTANT

PHASE ONE

I. A.M. Procedure

   A. Find out which pets are going home that day.

      1. Release date is the _____ line on boarding form.

      2. Most surgeries from previous day (not declaws).

   B. Rotate dogs into runs:

      1. Take tracking form or boarding form with pet and place on run door.

      2. Check form to find out correct diet. (Normally, one person does all feedings.)

         a. On boarding form, diet is found on middle of page. If that line is highlighted, it means the owner brought food from home which needs to be used.

         b. If not highlighted, use practice's food.

      3. Clean Compartments:

         a. Take out soiled papers and throw away.

         b. Wipe down all sides and bottom of compartment.

         c. Replace with 3 thickness newspapers to cover bottom.

         d. Remove water bowl.

      4. After dog has taken care of needs, place back into compartment.

      5. Clean run by using scrapers to pick up stools and then wash down run with hose.

      6. Continue this procedure until all dogs have been done.

   C. Cats

      1. Clean litter box. Note any abnormalities in stools or urine. If the cat was declawed the previous day, do not return litter box until that afternoon.

      2. If compartment is dirty, rotate cat to fresh compartment.

      3. Check form for proper diet. Feed all cats at the same time.

   D. Give fresh water to all pets.

   E. Assist the doctor with morning rounds when needed.

   F. After all pets have been taken care of, clean back area of practice.

      1. Vacuum entire back area.

      2. Spray down runs.

3. Mop Floors.

4. Change water in buckets, including mop bucket.

PHASE TWO

I. Getting pets ready to go home.

    A. If a TLC dog is going home, wash feet and stomach. Make sure animal is clean and odor-free. If the dog is to be given full a bath, wash it before the others.

    B. If non-TLC, place pet in hall compartment. If the dog is dirty or smells, rinse it off.

    C. If a boarder gets a full bath, proceed with normal bathing procedure. Do these baths before daily scheduled baths.

PHASE THREE

I. Baths

    A. Check file and tracking for any needed procedures. Be sure to check off the file and tracking form when completed.

    B. Check to see how many cat or dog baths are scheduled for the day and make up appropriate dip. Pay close attention to what kind of dip is being used in each bucket. DOG DIP WILL KILL CATS!

        1. For Dogs;

            a. Use dip.

            b. Dilute 1 oz. to 1 gallon of water.

        2. For Cats;

            a. Use dip.

            b. Dilute plunger to 1 quart of water.

    C. Get assistance.

        1. Comb out pet thoroughly.

        2. Trim nails.

        3. Place triple antibiotic ointment in both eyes.

        4. Do anal sacs (usually in tub).

    D. Place pet in tub and wet down hair coat. Wash head with baby shampoo.

        1. Dogs;

            a. Bathe body and rinse off.

            b. Dip dog in correct dip and be sure to saturate entire body. Do not get dip in eyes. Let set 5 minutes before rinsing.

    c. Use cream rinse and let sit for 5 minutes before rinsing.

  2. Cats;

    a. Bathe body in shampoo and rinse.

    b. Dip cat, saturating entire body. Do NOT get in eyes. Let sit for time indicated in product directions before rinsing.

    c. Use cream rinse on body and rinse after 5 minutes.

E. Towel dry then remove from tub and place on rack with dryer. Have dryer set on low or medium and monitor pet closely. Do NOT let pet overheat!

F. Clean up bath area and proceed with next bath.

G. After all baths are done;

  1. Comb out all TLC animals.

  2. Take other pets (in order of baths) out and comb. If not completely dry, blow dry.

PHASE FOUR

I. Constant monitoring of pets in back.

A. Continually check on pets in the back throughout the day.

  1. Clean any compartments that need it.

  2. Monitor pets waking up after surgery.

  3. Check to see that hospitalized animals have not vomited nor have diarrhea.

  4. Are fluids still running?

  5. If fluids have stopped or vomiting has occurred, inform a technician.

  6. IF SOMETHING JUST DOES NOT LOOK RIGHT - INFORM A TECHNICIAN OR DOCTOR!

B. When animals are discharged, clean compartment so it is ready for next animal.

PHASE FIVE

I. General maintenance of clinic.

A. After finishing all above duties, empty trash cans from office, bathroom, pharmacy, and exam rooms.

B. Sweep, then mop, reception room, office, pharmacy and exam rooms.

PHASE SIX

I. Launder towels and smocks

    A. Any dirty towels or smocks need to be washed, dried and then folded and put away.

PHASE SEVEN

I. Grocery shop for supplies.

    A. On Wednesdays, check list for needed supplies.

    B. Check supply of each item and if below stocked level, put on list.

    C. When list is complete, go to store.

    D. Be sure to bring back receipt.

VETERINARY RECEPTIONIST
PHASE TRAINING PROGRAM

PHASE ONE

I. Policies

    A. Personnel Paperwork

    B. Employee Handbook

    C. Dress Code

    D. Job Descriptions

    E. Job Priority List Review

II. The Mail

    A. Sorting Mail

    B. Exceptions

    C. Payments By Mail

    D. Out-going Mail

    E. Processing Held Checks

III. Filing

    A. Understanding the Filing System

    B. Pulling Files

    C. Alphabetize Files

    D. Do not file records that have lab work without notifying client.

    E. Multiple Places Where Records May Be Found

    F. All records not in use should be filed.

IV. Lab Work

    A. Lab work stored in green folder in file cabinet.

    B. Number is assigned to the lab work and recorded in the record.

    C. Lab work not filed until doctor has notified the client.

    D. After the above is done, lab work may be filed.

    E. Medical record may be filed.

V. Cleanliness of the Reception Area

    A. Reception area must be kept very clean at all times.

    B. Cleaning supplies are under the file cabinet.

    C. Call the ward manager for any "messes."

PHASE TWO

I. Opening

    A. Unlock doors, turn on lights, bring in newspaper.

    B. Turn on all computer terminals.

    C. Turn on main computer terminal in lab.

    D. Turn off phone recorder.

    E. Turn on lab equipment.

    F. Check appointment book with duplicate sheet.

    G. Double check to ensure that correct medical records are pulled for the day's appointments.

    H. Make sure front office and reception area are clean.

    I. Start coffee and make sure coffee area is well stocked and clean.

II. Admitting

    A. SMILE!

    B. Greet or acknowledge all clients as they walk in door.

    C. Check phone numbers for home and work.

    D. Check vaccine history and be sure the patient is current.

    E. If patient is eight years or older, we volunteer pre- surgical lab tests.

    F. Verify patient is coming in on an empty stomach.

    G. Keep only the animal; no jewelry or bedding.

    H. Inform client to contact the hospital after 3:00 p.m. to inquire of pet's well-being.

    I. If no questions, page the ward manager to admit patient.

III. Records

    A. Pull the patient medical record.

    B. Attach pink invoice, completely filled-out.

    C. Attach a report card.

    D. Attach client's check-in sheet.

    E. Make out appointment sheet.

    F. Put all the above into folder for that day.

IV. Appointments

    A. Medical record — record current date, weight and description of services necessary.

    B. Verify address and phone number.

    C. Check vaccine history to make sure the patient is current.

    D. Verify ALL information on any new client.

    E. Verify that pink sheet contains client's last name and patient name.

       1. When paperwork is complete, put on clipboard and up on counter.

       2. Signal exam-room filler.

    F. Confirm the Next Day's Appointments

       1. Mention the time, date and which doctor they will see.

       2. If it is a surgical appointment, remind client of all necessary pre-surgery instructions.

       3. Once the appointment has been confirmed, check the appointment book by the client's name.

       4. Indicate "N/A" by the client's name if there is no answer.

    G. Making Appointments

       1. Double check spelling of client's name.

       2. Write down the patient's name.

       3. Always double check day-time telephone number.

       4. Pull record while the client is on the phone to verify address and see what else animal is due for.

       5. Contact "no show" clients to reschedule their appointment.

V. Vaccines

    A. See Receptionist Information Box

       1. Know puppy and dog vaccination protocol.

       2. Know kitten and cat vaccination protocol.

       3. Study all other information contained within this box.

    B. Annual fecal checks are recommended on both dogs and cats

    C. Annual heartworm checks are recommended for dogs

VI. Petty Cash

    A. Petty cash is available for all employees as a loan or for small items to improve the hospital. Loans are not to exceed $10 per person per week.

PHASE THREE

I. Telephone Calls

    A. Answer the phone by the third ring.

    B. Always answer the phone by saying "Good morning/afternoon, ABC Veterinary Clinic. This is (name). May I help you?" Always use a friendly and pleasant voice and SMILE!

    C. If the call is to be returned, be very thorough in obtaining all the necessary information.

    D. Put message in the appropriate message box. No message should be taped to the counter top.

    E. Do not put the client on hold before asking their permission to do so. When returning to that call, thank them for holding and complete the call.

    F. All phone calls that are received between 8:00 a.m. and 12:00 noon will be returned at noon. All phone calls received between 12:00 noon and 3:00 p.m. will be returned at 3:00 p.m.

    G. Exceptions

        1. Family

        2. Other veterinarians

        3. Anything you consider to be an emergency

II. Invoicing

    A. Check medical record for services rendered.

    B. Check invoice to be sure that fees are listed for the appropriate services.

    C. If a recheck appointment is necessary, schedule it at this time.

    D. Bring up the invoicing screen on the computer

        1. Enter client number.

        2. Watch for stored services.

        3. Follow instructions on screen.

        4. Include all services on invoice.

        5. Before concluding, check to see if client needs anything else.

        6. Check to see if there is a discount.

        7. Make sure client has medicine dispensed.

        8. Conclude invoice.

        9. Method of payment and amount.

        10. Check for previous balance.

III. Deceased Pet Records

    A. Inactive patient records

    B. Remove code under patient file in the computer.

    C. Put a yellow dot on the patient file.

    D. Put the card in the folder for a sympathy letter.

    E. Card is filed in deceased animal file.

IV. Prescriptions

    A. Telephone request for refill

        1. Get the name of client and pet

        2. Pull medical record.

        3. Get approval from the doctor.

        4. Record on the medical card.

        5. Put record and a note in the pharmacy to notify the technician when the client will pick it up.

        6. Once the prescription is filled, the file and the medication will be placed in the "reading-station" box.

        7. NO MEDICINE IS DISPENSED UNLESS APPROVED BY A DOCTOR!

        8. Exceptions are maintenance drugs which are listed on the upper left of the record.

        9. When the client comes in for the prescription, always double check the dosage to ensure that they are giving the medication correctly.

    B. If a client walks-in for medication

        1. First, ask the client if they previously called it in.

        2. If they haven't called it in, then repeat the process of the telephone request — Do this in an expedient manner!

V. Back-Up

    A. Follow written instructions in green notebook.

    B. Back-up should be done daily between 12:00 noon and 3:00 p.m.

    C. All terminals should be backed out to the initial log-in screen before starting back-up.

    D. Double back-up is done on Wednesday.

    E. An extra back-up is also done once a month.

    F. Check previous day's record to find out which tape to use.

    G. Tapes and diskettes are kept in the doctor's office.

VI. Discharging Patients

    A. In-Hospital Patients

        1. Clients are encouraged to call after 3:00 p.m. to inquire about the health and well-being of their pet.

        2. Always check patient report form.

        3. Inform the client that the hospital has visiting hours which are from 10:00 a.m. to 11:30 a.m. and between 4:00 p.m. and 6:00 p.m.

    B. Follow invoicing instructions.

    C. If vaccines were given, update reminder column on medical record.

    D. If spayed or neutered, indicate on the medical record.

    E. Make recheck appointment, if necessary.

    F. If there is a question regarding the bill, have the client speak with the practice manager.

    G. All bills must be paid in full.

    H. Held checks are acceptable up to two months. Anything beyond that should be discussed first with the practice manager.

    I. If there are any further problems, consult with the practice manager.

    J. If there is a black dot in the corner of the record, then this would indicate that there was a bad debt or trouble collecting in the past.

    K. Computer flags all have a meaning and should be dealt with before continuing invoicing on that client. Again, check with the practice manager.

VII. Closing

    A. At doctor's request, put on recording machine and flip switch for phones.

    B Lock both doors.

    C. Clean reception room and front desk area.

    D. Dust the tables.

    E. Turn off the scale.

    F. Remove invoicing paper and put in the white paper.

    G. Run and close the books.

    I. Turn off all the computers.

    J. Replace invoicing paper and reset printer.

    K. Clean reception area.

    L. If a maintenance person is not in, then turn off the lights and lock all doors.

    M. Make sure back door is securely locked.

EXAM ROOM TECHNICIAN
PHASE TRAINING PROGRAM

PHASE ONE

I. Policies

    A. Personnel Paperwork

    B. Employee Handbook

    C. Dress Code

    D. Job Descriptions

PHASE TWO

I. Set Up Lab

    A. Uncover microscope, get out book.

    B. Plug in and turn on equipment.

    C. Take tests out of refrigerator.

    D. Take tray out of refrigerator—put in laboratory.

PHASE THREE

I. Client Check-In

    A. Routine Appointments

        1. Escort client from waiting room into exam room.

        2. Review vaccinations needed.

        3. HW test needed? Preventative?

        4. Problems or questions for the doctor?

        5. Take animal back for HW and NT.

    B. Surgeries, Dentistries

        1. Client already in room.

        2. Confirm procedure to be done. Give info sheet.

        3. Bloodwork required for animals over 5 yrs; recommend for anyone else.

        4. HW test required for all surgeries if born before 11/1 of same year.

        5. Any other problems?

        6. Obtain phone number where can be reached and authorization signature.

        7. Inform client appt/go procedure.

    C. Non-routine Appointments

        1. Reason for appointment.

      2. Temp if animal is ill.

      3. Ask questions, if have time (see list).

II. After Client Check-In

    A. File on pharmacy counter with doctor's clip.

    B. Locate doctor if necessary.

    C. Put vacs/rabies tag (if needed) on file.

    D. Start fecal.

      1. Write patient's name and room number in lab book. Label tube or mark number in centrifuge corresponding to patient's name.

      2. Centrifuge for 5 minutes.

      3. Record results in lab book.

    E. Run heartworm test

      1. Patient's name in lab book.

      2. Initial snap test with pet's first/last name.

      3. Record results in lab book.

III. Assist doctor in exam room, if necessary

PHASE FOUR

I. Other Lab Work - Fecals, Bloodwork

    A. Daily

      1. Clean floor.

      2. Clean table and counter.

      3. Turn off light.

      4. Shut door.

    B. Weekly

      1. Stock.

      2. Clean all areas.

      3. Vacuum seat.

II. Fill Prescriptions

    A. If in doubt about a refill, check with the doctor.

    B. Labels are in pharmacy and are to include:

      1. Patient's name.

    2. Date.

    3. Dosage.

    4. Doctor's name.

    5. Expiration date.

    6. Name of drug.

    7. Quantity.

    8. Special instructions given by doctor.

PHASE FIVE

I. Grooming List

  A. Include:

    1. Patient's name.

    2. What is to be done.

    3. Any Rx refills.

    4. Patient's weight.

    5. Time of pick-up.

    6. Phone number where owner can be reached.

  B. Label with appropriate doctor.

  C. Set up vaccines, HW syringes, fecal tubes - put in file.

  D. Fill out TS, yellow sheet, examination sheet - put in file.

VETERINARY ASSISTANT
PHASE TRAINING PROGRAM

PHASE ONE

I. Interaction with Patients and Clients

    A. How to Communicate with Patients

        1. Treat the animals as you would your own.

        2. Animals respond more to love than tolerance.

        3. Always respect them.

        4. Greet them like a friend.

    B. How to Communicate with Clients

        1. Make them feel at home.

        2. Show them that you care.

        3. Listen carefully to what they say.

        4. Always talk to them and smile!

    C. Providing Assistance to Patients and Clients

        1. Offer to carry items.

        2. Provide answers or help to get an answer.

II. Animal Care Protocol

    A. Proper Care of Boarding and Hospitalized Patients

        1. Know proper way to read and fill out all information in the boarding and treatment book.

        2. Be aware of any special needs of the patient.

        3. "X" off in record when services/procedures are complete.

    B. What to Provide for Patients

        1. Proper food, taking note of special diets

        2. Water at all times

        3. Comfortable and appropriate bedding

        4. Love and attention to relieve stress

    C. Proper Walking Techniques

        1. Walk animals at least three times daily.

        2. Walk in the appropriate areas.

        3. Take note of any physical problems that may affect walking.

            a. ruptured discs, back problems, etc.

       b. blindness

       c. inability to hold urine for long periods of time

    4. Proper length of time for walks

III. Animal Handling Techniques

  A. Restraining Patients for Exams

    1. Realize the client/owner will be in the room.

    2. Use precautions when necessary.

    3. Never be overconfident about an animal.

    4. Know the doctor's routine.

       a. position of the animal (head away or towards the doctor, etc.)

       b. when to hold tighter

  B. Restraining the Patient for Sample Collection

    1. Use muzzles and/or cat bags when needed.

    2. Hold tightly without harming the animal.

    3. Be gentle.

    4. Know different techniques.

       a. holding off a front leg (dog or cat)

       b. holding off a back leg (dog or cat)

       c. holding large and small dogs

       d. scruffing a cat

       e. holding for use of the jugular vein

IV. Performing Baths and Dips

  A. Shampoo/Dip Orientation

    1. Use of different types

    2. Precautions of different types

  B. Bathing Techniques

    1. Precautions

       a. protection of eyes

       b. never leave the animal

    2. Lathering and rinsing

    3. Timing of the shampoo

  C. Drying Techniques

    1. Proper level on the dryer

2. Timing of the dryer

D. Performing nail trims, ear cleanings, shaving,, etc.

E. Being Aware of Your Patient

    1. Notice if the animal has any problems

        a. lumps

        b. bite wounds

        c. ticks

        d. skin or hair problems

        e. eye or ear problems

F. Be Able to Recommend Products for Future Use

PHASE TWO

I. Hospital Maintenance

    A. Emptying Trash Cans

    B. Vacuuming and Mopping Hospital Floors

    C. Overall Appearance of Hospital

        1. Windows

        2. Benches

        3. Walls

        4. Cabinets

    D. Maintenance of Public Restroom

        1. Cleanliness

        2. Fully supplied

    E. Maintenance of Exterior Hospital

        1. Garbage placed in trash bins

        2. Front area free of animal waste

II. Ward Maintenance

    A. Cleaning Kennels

        1. Using proper solutions

            a. regular cleaning

            b. infectious cages

    B. Cleaning Supplies and Location

    C. Protocol for Cleaning Contaminated Areas

    D. Protocol for Cleaning Isolation Areas

E. Proper Disposal of Contaminated Items

    1. Sharps containers

    2. Hazardous liquids and solids

    3. Bodies

III. Cleaning Exam Rooms

  A. Vacuuming or Sweeping Floors (mop if necessary)

  B. Wipe Counter Tops, Sink and Table

    1. Routine cleaning between patients

    2. Weekly cleaning

  C. Clean Dirtied Equipment (combs, ear cones, etc.)

  D. Tidy Equipment

    1. Make sure all instruments are available.

    2. Remove all used syringes and other items used before.

  E. Straighten Reading Materials and Informational Books

  F. Empty Trash Can if Needed

  G. Deodorize If Necessary

IV. Autoclave Protocol

  A. Proper Cleaning of Instruments

  B. Preparation of Packs

  C. Preparation of Individual Instruments

  D. Proper Labeling

  E. Use of Autoclave

V. Maintenance of Surgical/Hospital Equipment

  A. Cleaning of Anesthesia Machines

    1. Hoses

    2. Valves

    3. Masks

    4. Bags

  B. Charging of Monitors

  C. Cleaning of Table and Light

PHASE THREE

I. X-Ray Orientation

    A. Read and Sign Off on Radiology Hospital Manual

    B. Issue Radiation Badge

    C. Demonstration of X-Ray Equipment and Proper Use

II. X-Ray Taking Techniques

    A. Proper Positioning of Patients

    B. Explanation of Anatomy and Views

        1. V/D, LAT, A/P, etc.

        2. Abdomen, cranial, lumbar, etc.

    C. X-Ray Log

III. Developing X-Rays

    A. X-Ray Room Explanation

        1. Processor

        2. Folders

        3. Film and cassettes

    B. Use of the Developer

    C. Preparing Cassettes and Film

    D. Preparing Folders

IV. Filing X-Rays

    A. Explanation of Filing System

    B. Location of Files, Films and Relevant Supplies

    C. Distinction of Wildlife Files

PHASE FOUR

I. Exam Room Handler Protocol

    A. Outline of Duties

    B. Flow of Outpatient Appointments

    C. Technician Support for Technicians and Doctors

        1. Collection of samples

        2. Restraint for both examinations and treatments

II. Assisting Technicians with the Collection of Samples

   A. Necessary Equipment

      1. Syringes

      2. Tubes

      3. Solutions

      4. Swabs

      5. Fecal loops

   B. Proper Restraint Techniques

III. Product Orientation

   A. Flea and Tick Problems

   B. Heartworm Preventatives

   C. Dietary/Nutritional Products

   D. Accessories

   E. Shampoos and Conditioners

ASSISTANT MANAGER / BOOKKEEPER EVALUATION

Name _____ Date _____

Date of last review _____ Date of Employment _____

Person preparing review _____

RATING GUIDE

U	Unsatisfactory	0 points
N	Needs Improvement	1 point
S	Satisfactory	2 points
A	Above Average	3 points
E	Excellent	4 points

ACCURACY AND THOROUGHNESS

Does employee have a clear understanding of the job description and duties?

Rating ____ **Comments** _____

Does the employee have a clear understanding of the clinic philosophy and a thorough understanding of the mission statement?

Rating ____ **Comments** _____

COOPERATION

Does the employee get along with fellow employees?

Rating ____ **Comments** _____

Does the employee take direction and criticism well?

Rating ____ **Comments** _____

Is the employee punctual and dependable?

Rating ____ **Comments** _____

Does the employee spend time productively?

Rating ____ **Comments** _____

Does the employee keep the work area clean and neat?

Rating ____ **Comments** _____

Does the employee present the proper appearance (neat and adhering to dress code)?

Rating ____ **Comments** _____

COOPERATION *(Continued)*

Is the employee flexible with scheduling and fills in when needed?

Rating ____ **Comments** _____

Does the employee understand basic computer concepts and is able to follow directions in computer use, back up, and trouble shooting? Does the employee enter information correctly?

Rating ____ **Comments** _____

ACCOUNTING/BOOKKEEPING

Prepares and issues financial statements (income statements and balance sheets).

Rating ____ **Comments** _____

Assesses financial position of practice.

Rating ____ **Comments** _____

Reduces accounts receivable and shows proficiency at collection procedures.

Rating ____ **Comments** _____

Is efficient at problem solving.

Rating ____ **Comments** _____

Prepares financial budget.

Rating ____ **Comments** _____

PUBLIC RELATIONS

Uses appropriate interpersonal techniques when interacting with clients.

Rating ____ **Comments** _____

PURCHASING

Negotiates optimal prices.

Rating ____ **Comments** _____

PRACTICE MANAGEMENT

Controls expenses of practice to best of ability.

Rating ____ **Comments** _____

Handles paperwork efficiently.

Rating ____ **Comments** _____

Sets priorities, budgets time well, and avoids unnecessary expenditure of time on non-productive tasks.

Rating ____ **Comments** _____

Promotes practice well.

Rating ____ **Comments** _____

PRACTICE MANAGEMENT (Continued)

Keeps current in field by reading journals and participates in continuing education.

Rating ____ **Comments** _____

Additional Comments:

_____

_____

_____

_____

_____

_____

Action Recommended:

_____

_____

_____

_____

_____

_____

Employee Signature: _____

Date: _____

Associate Evaluation Form

Name _____ Date _____

Date of last review _____ Date of Employment _____

Associate Evaluation Form

Grading

1 - Needs improvement

2 - Adequate

3 - Very Good

4 - Excellent

Personal and General Skills

_____ Always looks professional, clean, and neatly groomed

_____ Wears name tags and a clean white jacket

_____ Keeps a positive attitude

_____ Gets along with staff and doctors

_____ Does not get too personally involved with staff

_____ Punctual and dependable

_____ Is neat and uses a "clean as you go" philosophy

Communication

_____ Explains instructions and diagnoses well to clients in easy to understand terms. Avoids overuse of medical terms

_____ Gives accurate estimates and obtains permission from owners before treatment or surgery is begun

_____ Teaches staff about procedures and philosophy

_____ Has good follow-through concerning client call backs and makes appropriate comments in records concerning callbacks

_____ Considers the client's emotional interest as well as the pet's comfort when making a decision

_____ Instills confidence to staff and clients

Surgical Skills

_____ Has a good understanding of anesthesia, drugs, and equipment

_____ Is considerate of pain and comfort of patients

_____ Dresses appropriately for surgery and uses aseptic technique

_____ Completes surgery in a reasonable amount of time

_____ Is not wasteful of surgical or anesthesia supplies

_____ Has a good knowledge of anatomy when doing non-routine surgical procedures

_____ Makes an attempt to improve deficiency areas of surgery by practice on cadavers or asking for help in difficult surgeries

_____ Charges appropriately for surgery time

Record Keeping

_____ SOAPs records accurately

_____ Communicates with the other doctor(s) through notations on the record

_____ Updates Anesthesia/Surgery Log and controlled substance log in a timely fashion

_____ Fills out laboratory submission sheet accurately

_____ Updates treatment records on a timely basis

Examinations

_____ Is prompt for exam visits

_____ Spends sufficient time with each patient/client

_____ Is productive with time and income with each visit

_____ Gives a technically good physical exam to every patient and charges accordingly

_____ Uses visual aids to explain points to clients

_____ Obtains owner's permission and gives estimate before initiating treatment

_____ Allows clients to make decision concerning whether they want service suggested. Is not preoccupied with "X-raying the client's pocketbook" and is thorough in suggestions of services needed

_____ Sees and charges appropriately for emergencies

_____ Stays very accessible when on emergency call

Management and Marketing

_____ Has reasonable understanding of overhead cost and considers ways to increase income

_____ Sends employees who have concerns or criticisms to the Practice Manager rather than getting involved

_____ Maintains inventory well and makes effort to write down short supply stock

_____ Uses free materials to save hospital money as opposed to using supplies that hospital pays for

_____ Makes an effort to learn more about the business portion of the veterinary practice

_____ Supports the need to do target marketing as well as internal and external marketing

_____ Maintains a good control on accounts receivables and has a good understanding that all services have a fee attached

_____ Is consciously aware of the exterior and interior appearance of the building. Using caution with chain leashes and equipment, etc. to save hospital repairs

_____ Notices exterior grounds daily and cleans up trash or fecal material from the yard and parking lot

_____ Periodically walks in the front door as a client to make sure first impression is always excellent

_____ Shows interest and asks questions concerning management and marketing of services

Comments and Major Improvements Noted

_____

_____

_____

_____

_____

Goals to be Accomplished During the Following Year:

_____

_____

_____

_____

_____

EMPLOYEE REVIEW FORM

Name _____ Date _____

Classification _____ Score _____

Attitude and Interest

_____ Enthusiastic

_____ Interested

_____ Average

_____ Somewhat indifferent

_____ Other: _____

Adaptability

_____ Adjusts easily-very well liked

_____ Good team worker

_____ Cooperates satisfactorily

Has difficulty working with others

_____ Other: _____

Ability to Learn

_____ Grasps ideas very quickly

_____ Above average

_____ Average

_____ Rather slow to learn

_____ Other: _____

Quality of Work

_____ Excellent

_____ Above average

_____ Average

_____ Below average

_____ Other: _____

Quantity of Work

_____ Unusually high output

_____ Above average

_____ Average

_____ Less than expected

_____ Other: _____

Dependability

_____ Entirely dependable

_____ Requires little supervision

_____ Satisfactory

_____ Sometimes neglectful or forgetful

_____ Other: _____

Housekeeping

_____ Cleans whatever needs to be cleaned without prompting

_____ Notices most things that need to be corrected

_____ Cleans only the most obvious problems

_____ Needs improvement

_____ Other: _____

Initiative

_____ Takes hold readily

_____ Above average

_____ Goes ahead reasonably well

_____ Somewhat lacking

_____ Other: _____

Judgement

_____ Displays excellent common sense

_____ Usually does the right thing

_____ Ordinary

_____ Occasionally uses poor judgement

_____ Other: _____

Creativity

_____ Exceptional original thinking and follow-through

_____ Occasional creativeness

_____ Average

_____ Mediocre

_____ Other: _____

Industriousness

_____ Works steadily

_____ Usually working

_____ Works as steadily as average

_____ Does not work steadily

_____ Other: _____

Attendance

Regular _____   Irregular _____

Punctuality

Regular _____   Irregular _____

In summation, general appraisal of individual's performance for future success:

Outstanding _____   Very good _____   Satisfactory _____   Mediocre _____
Other _____

Additional Comments:

_____

_____

_____

_____

_____

_____

_____

HOSPITAL EVALUATION

Please use this form to evaluate the ABC Veterinary Hospital and its management. Please answer honestly and know that your answers and comments will remain anonymous. Thank you for your time and cooperation.

RATING GUIDE

Unsatisfactory	0 points
Needs Improvement	1 point
Satisfactory	2 points
Above Average	3 points
Excellent	4 points

1. Supervises staff personnel and follows up on disciplinary procedures.

   Rating ___ **Comments** _____

2. Maintains employment policies and hospital manual, updating when needed.

   Rating ___ **Comments** _____

3. Conducts productive staff meetings at regular intervals. Departmental, general and social meetings with published agendas.

   Rating ___ **Comments** _____

4. Management maintains employee motivation to the best of their ability.

   Rating ___ **Comments** _____

5. Implements new ideas.

   Rating ___ **Comments** _____

6. Promotes the practice.

   Rating ___ **Comments** _____

7. Does employment reviews in a professional, timely fashion.

   Rating ___ **Comments** _____

8. Develops and accomplishes a practice marketing program.

   Rating ___ **Comments** _____

9. Schedules and conducts hospital tours.

   Rating ___ **Comments** _____

10. Enhances public perception of the practice.

   Rating ___ **Comments** _____

11. Delegates responsibility well.

   Rating ___ **Comments** _____

12. Demonstrates effective communication skills.

   Rating ___ **Comments** _____

13. Acknowledges outstanding work.

   Rating ___ **Comments** _____

14. Actively listens to staff.

   Rating ___ **Comments** _____

15. What do you consider to be the quality of veterinary services provided to clients?

   Rating ___ **Comments** _____

16. In your estimation, what would be the rating given by clients regarding the value and quality of veterinary services rendered within the practice?

   Rating ___ **Comments** _____

17. How happy are you in your present job and position?

   Rating ___ **Comments** _____

18. How well do you feel that management communicates with you?

   Rating ___ **Comments** _____

19. Do you feel that you are adequately compensated for the work you do?

   Rating ___ **Comments** _____

20. How effective is management at providing feedback in regards to the work that you do?

   Rating ___ **Comments** _____

21. How open is management to new ideas and suggestions?

   Rating ___ **Comments** _____

Please feel free to provide additional feedback below. Thank you!

_____

_____

_____

_____

ATTENDANT EVALUATION FORM

Name _____ Date _____

Date of last review _____ Date of Employment _____

Person preparing review _____

RATING GUIDE

U	Unsatisfactory	0 points
N	Needs Improvement	1 point
S	Satisfactory	2 points
A	Above Average	3 points
E	Excellent	4 points

HANDLING ANIMALS

Safe and effective handler

Rating ____ **Comments** _____

Able to restrain animals for procedures

Rating ____ **Comments** _____

Shows gentleness and compassion

Rating ____ **Comments** _____

CLEANING

Keeps wards and cages clean

Rating ____ **Comments** _____

Keeps litter pans clean

Rating ____ **Comments** _____

Keeps front office clean

Rating ____ **Comments** _____

Keeps parking lot clean

Rating ____ **Comments** _____

Keeps animals clean while kenneled

Rating ____ **Comments** _____

PROTOCOL

Knows how to admit animals

Rating ___ **Comments** _____

Knows how to release animals

Rating ___ **Comments** _____

Knows how to assist in emergencies

Rating ___ **Comments** _____

Familiar with inventory systems

Rating ___ **Comments** _____

Able to stock front office/treatment room

Rating ___ **Comments** _____

Opens/closes kennel as directed

Rating ___ **Comments** _____

Does laundry duty

Rating **Comments**

GROOMING

Able to give bath/dip properly

Rating ___ **Comments** _____

Able to flush ears properly

Rating ___ **Comments** _____

Able to clip nails

Rating ___ **Comments** _____

Able to check anal sacs

Rating ___ **Comments** _____

Recognizes fleas/flea dirt

Rating ___ **Comments** _____

FEEDING/MEDICATION

Able to medicate animals as directed

Rating ___ **Comments** _____

Familiar with special diets

Rating ___ **Comments** _____

Notifies doctor promptly of appetite problems

Rating ___ **Comments** _____

Knows feeding procedures

Rating ___ **Comments** _____

Keeps animals watered

Rating ___ **Comments** _____

VETERINARY APTITUDE

Recognizes signs of illness in animals

Rating ___ **Comments** _____

Promptly notifies doctors of problems

Rating ___ **Comments** _____

Aids in generating lab results

Rating ___ **Comments** _____

Aids in treatments

Rating ___ **Comments** _____

Technician duties being developed

Rating ___ **Comments** _____

PERSONAL

Shows initiative in finding things to do during idle times

Rating ___ **Comments** _____

Adheres to the dress code

Rating ___ **Comments** _____

Appears well groomed

Rating ___ **Comments** _____

Professional behavior

Rating ___ **Comments** _____

COMMENTS:

_____

_____

_____

_____

_____

_____

I have discussed this evaluation with _____ *and understand my responsibilities.*

Signed: _____

Date: _____

Effectiveness Evaluation:

Veterinary Practice Manager

Name _____ Date _____

Date of last review _____ Date of Employment _____

Evaluated by _____

Practice Manager's Effectiveness Evaluation

Grading

5 - Highly effective

4 - Effective

3 - Average

2 - Improvement needed

1 - Great improvement needed

N/A - Not applicable

Practice Manager's Rating		Practitioner's Rating
SECTION ONE - FEES		
5 4 3 2 1 N/A	Develops cost estimates	5 4 3 2 1 N/A
5 4 3 2 1 N/A	Deals with financial problems with clients successfully	5 4 3 2 1 N/A
5 4 3 2 1 N/A	Periodically reviews and establishes a new fee schedule	5 4 3 2 1 N/A
5 4 3 2 1 N/A	Strives to help practice reach full profitability potential	5 4 3 2 1 N/A
SECTION TWO - PERSONNEL		
5 4 3 2 1 N/A	Hires staff	5 4 3 2 1 N/A
5 4 3 2 1 N/A	Manages staff	5 4 3 2 1 N/A
5 4 3 2 1 N/A	Formulates job descriptions	5 4 3 2 1 N/A
5 4 3 2 1 N/A	Schedules staff	5 4 3 2 1 N/A
5 4 3 2 1 N/A	Develops work plans for specially assigned projects	5 4 3 2 1 N/A
5 4 3 2 1 N/A	Creates and utilizes incentives for high performance	5 4 3 2 1 N/A
5 4 3 2 1 N/A	Recognizes and rewards improved and outstanding performance	5 4 3 2 1 N/A
5 4 3 2 1 N/A	Motivates staff	5 4 3 2 1 N/A
5 4 3 2 1 N/A	Conducts performance reviews	5 4 3 2 1 N/A
5 4 3 2 1 N/A	Solves problems	5 4 3 2 1 N/A
5 4 3 2 1 N/A	Sets salaries	5 4 3 2 1 N/A
5 4 3 2 1 N/A	Mediates staff conflict	5 4 3 2 1 N/A
5 4 3 2 1 N/A	Disciplines staff	5 4 3 2 1 N/A
5 4 3 2 1 N/A	Discharges staff appropriately when necessary	5 4 3 2 1 N/A
5 4 3 2 1 N/A	Delegates responsibility	5 4 3 2 1 N/A
5 4 3 2 1 N/A	Supervises staff training and development	5 4 3 2 1 N/A

SECTION THREE - PURCHASING

5 4 3 2 1 N/A Negotiates optimal prices	5 4 3 2 1 N/A
5 4 3 2 1 N/A Arranges bulk and group purchases	5 4 3 2 1 N/A
5 4 3 2 1 N/A Keeps abreast of new products	5 4 3 2 1 N/A
5 4 3 2 1 N/A Keeps abreast of new pharmaceuticals	5 4 3 2 1 N/A
5 4 3 2 1 N/A Meets with drug company representatives	5 4 3 2 1 N/A
5 4 3 2 1 N/A Controls inventory	5 4 3 2 1 N/A

SECTION FOUR - ACCOUNTING/BOOKKEEPING

5 4 3 2 1 N/A Prepares and issues financial statements (income statements, balance sheets and departmentalized profit/loss statements)	5 4 3 2 1 N/A
5 4 3 2 1 N/A Assesses the financial position of the practice	5 4 3 2 1 N/A
5 4 3 2 1 N/A Plans for the growth of the practice	5 4 3 2 1 N/A
5 4 3 2 1 N/A Reduces accounts receivable	5 4 3 2 1 N/A
5 4 3 2 1 N/A Shows proficiency at collection procedures	5 4 3 2 1 N/A

SECTION FIVE - ORGANIZATION OF PRACTICE

5 4 3 2 1 N/A Maintains positive practice environment	5 4 3 2 1 N/A
5 4 3 2 1 N/A Is efficient and fair at problem solving	5 4 3 2 1 N/A

SECTION SIX - PUBLIC RELATIONS

5 4 3 2 1 N/A Uses appropriate interpersonal techniques when interacting with clients	5 4 3 2 1 N/A
5 4 3 2 1 N/A Establishes a volunteer program	5 4 3 2 1 N/A
5 4 3 2 1 N/A Develops hospital brochure/folder	5 4 3 2 1 N/A
5 4 3 2 1 N/A Involves practice in public speaking opportunities	5 4 3 2 1 N/A
5 4 3 2 1 N/A Initiates new programs	5 4 3 2 1 N/A

SECTION SEVEN - BENEFIT PROGRAMS

5 4 3 2 1 N/A Evaluates and establishes new benefit programs	5 4 3 2 1 N/A
5 4 3 2 1 N/A Appraises benefit programs and administers them	5 4 3 2 1 N/A

SECTION EIGHT - GROWTH PLANNING

5 4 3 2 1 N/A Prepares financial budget	5 4 3 2 1 N/A
5 4 3 2 1 N/A Assists in future planning and directions	5 4 3 2 1 N/A
5 4 3 2 1 N/A Keeps current in field (reads journals and attends seminars)	5 4 3 2 1 N/A

SECTION NINE - OVERALL PRACTICE MANAGEMENT

5 4 3 2 1 N/A	Controls expenses of practice to the best of ability	5 4 3 2 1 N/A
5 4 3 2 1 N/A	Handles paperwork efficiently	5 4 3 2 1 N/A
5 4 3 2 1 N/A	Controls personal emotions well	5 4 3 2 1 N/A
5 4 3 2 1 N/A	Sets priorities and budgets time well	5 4 3 2 1 N/A
5 4 3 2 1 N/A	Avoids unnecessary expenditure of time on non-productive tasks	5 4 3 2 1 N/A
5 4 3 2 1 N/A	Promotes practice well	5 4 3 2 1 N/A

SECTION TEN - COMMENTS AND RECOMMENDATIONS

_____

_____

_____

_____

_____

Partner Performance

Self Evaluation

Name: _____

Date: _____

Evaluation Period: From _____ To _____

Instructions: Please provide your honest, most objective assessment of your performance. Please return the completed from to _____ no later than _____, 19___.

Please retain a copy of this form for your records.

Ratings:

5   OUTSTANDING (Realistically, as good as we could hope or expect.)

4   VERY GOOD (Generally satisfactory – what we could expect from a partner in our practice.)

3   GOOD (Reasonable performance – would be acceptable but not worthy of merit.)

2   FAIR (Below our acceptance level for a partner in our practice.)

1   POOR (Probably has a negative impact on other partners, staff or clients.)

N   NOT APPLICABLE or I Cannot Really Judge This

SECTION ONE

With a pencil or pen, darken one rating for each item listed. If you would like to explain any answer, circle the number and use the space provided in Section Two of this form for your explanation, making sure to reference the appropriate letter and number for each (example: "A, #3").

Rating

A.   Personal Qualities

1. Gets Things Done (a "Doer") — Accomplishes tasks	5 4 3 2 1 [N]
2. Enthusiasm, Positive Nature, Upbeat – "Can Do" Attitude	5 4 3 2 1 [N]
3. Leadership (Ability to Motivate Others)	5 4 3 2 1 [N]
4. Temperament (Easygoing versus Volatile)	5 4 3 2 1 [N]
5. Honest, Trustworthy, Moral Character	5 4 3 2 1 [N]
6. Cooperative – "Team Player" versus "Selfish"	5 4 3 2 1 [N]
7. Work Ethic (Effort, Hard Work, Commitment)	5 4 3 2 1 [N]
8. Delegates Appropriately and Follows Up	5 4 3 2 1 [N]
9. Communication and Presentation Skills	5 4 3 2 1 [N]
10. Decision Making, Common Sense, Judgement	5 4 3 2 1 [N]

B. Business Development and Practice Promotion

1. Develops Practice Name in the Community	5 4 3 2 1 [N]
2. Generates Appropriate Type and Quantity of New Business	5 4 3 2 1 [N]

3. Active with Referral Sources, Clients, and/or   5   4   3   2   1   [N]
   Business Leaders

4. Ability to Sell (Sales Skills)   5   4   3   2   1   [N]

5. Provides Ideas and Activities Designed to Generate   5   4   3   2   1   [N]
   Additional Revenue

C. Client Service

1. Provides Innovative and Timely Service to Clients   5   4   3   2   1   [N]

2. Attentiveness and Responsiveness to Clients' Needs   5   4   3   2   1   [N]
   (Develops Confidence)

3. Provides Quality Service on a Timely Basis   5   4   3   2   1   [N]

D. Cooperation and Compliance With Practice Policies and Procedures

1. Adherence to Practice Policies   5   4   3   2   1   [N]

2. Adherence to Practice Quality Control System   5   4   3   2   1   [N]

3. Relationship with Administrative Staff and Associates   5   4   3   2   1   [N]

4. Participation in Practice Functions and/or In-house   5   4   3   2   1   [N]
   Training Programs

E. Performance of Management/Administrative Functions

1. Management of Practice Activities   5   4   3   2   1   [N]

2. Administrative or Personnel Related Activities   5   4   3   2   1   [N]

3. Other Activities (Where the Practice or Partners Can Be   5   4   3   2   1   [N]
   Considered "The Client")

F. Profitability Factors

1. Gross Fees (Revenue Produced) From My Clients   5   4   3   2   1   [N]

2. Number of Professional Transactions   5   4   3   2   1   [N]

3. Average Client Charge – Client Profitability   5   4   3   2   1   [N]

4. Receivable Collection Effectiveness and Bad Debts   5   4   3   2   1   [N]

5. Retention of Profitable Clients   5   4   3   2   1   [N]

SECTION TWO

Use the space below for comments regarding Section One. Circle the number in Section One above and note the appropriate letter and number next to each comment or explanation. (example: "A, #3, Leadership skills")

_____

_____

_____

_____

_____

_____

_____

_____

_____

_____

_____

_____

_____

_____

SECTION THREE

A   List your goals for the past 12 months. You may use the space provided below or attach your existing list. Evaluate your performance in regard to these goals.

_____

_____

_____

_____

_____

_____

_____

_____

_____

_____

_____

_____

_____

_____

_____

_____

_____

_____

_____

_____

_____

_____

_____

B.   Provide any other comments regarding your appraisal of your year's
     performance.

_____

_____

_____

_____

_____

_____

_____

_____

C.   List your goals for the next 12 months in the space below. If possible, they
     should be:

   1.   Objectively <u>measurable</u>.

   2.   As specific as possible.

   3.   Dependent on you rather than other people.

   4.   Attainable (i.e. realistic, but challenging).

   5.   Appropriate for your personality and responsibilities.

_____

_____

_____

_____

_____

_____

_____

_____

_____

_____

C. Goals for the Next 12 Months (Continued)

_____

_____

_____

_____

_____

_____

_____

_____

_____

SECTION FOUR

Do you have any additional suggestions, recommendations or comments? **This is very important**.

_____

_____

_____

_____

_____

_____

_____

_____

_____

_____

_____

_____

_____

RECEPTIONIST EVALUATION

Name _____ Date _____

Date of last review _____ Date of Employment _____

Person preparing review _____

RATING GUIDE

U	Unsatisfactory	0 points
N	Needs Improvement	1 point
S	Satisfactory	2 points
A	Above Average	3 points
E	Excellent	4 points

I. People Skills

Does employee help clients at the front desk quickly and cheerfully?

Rating ___ **Comments** _____

Does the employee answer phone promptly? Give the proper impression on the telephone?

Rating ___ **Comments** _____

Does the employee show "grace under pressure"? How does the employee handle the front desk when it gets busy?

Rating ___ **Comments** _____

How well does the employee remember names (both clients and pets)?

Rating ___ **Comments** _____

How does the employee relate to pets?

Rating ___ **Comments** _____

Does the employee convey warmth and concern?

Rating ___ **Comments** _____

II. Accuracy, Thoroughness

Is employee neat and accurate in record-keeping, making appointments, etc.? Is employee accurate with transactions?

Rating ___ **Comments** _____

Is the employee well versed in information to give clients (vaccination schedules, parasite prevention, etc.)?

Rating ___ **Comments** _____

Does the employee make efforts to educate the client with regard to parasite control, etc.?

Rating ___ **Comments** _____

III. Productivity

Does employee spend time productively?

Rating ___ **Comments** _____

Does employee look for additional tasks?

Rating ___ **Comments** _____

Does employee have suggestions for improvements?

Rating ___ **Comments** _____

Does employee accept responsibility well?

Rating ___ **Comments** _____

Does the employee tire easily, take excessive breaks?

Rating ___ **Comments** _____

Does employee perform housekeeping duties, keep work area neat and clean?

Rating ___ **Comments** _____

Does employee work well without supervision?

Rating ___ **Comments** _____

Does employee present the proper appearance (neat, in uniform)?

Rating ___ **Comments** _____

IV. Dependability, Cooperation

Is the employee punctual and dependable?

Rating ___ **Comments** _____

Is employee flexible with scheduling, fills in when needed?

Rating ___ **Comments** _____

Does employee get along well with fellow employees?

Rating ___ **Comments** _____

Has employee taken initiative to learn others' jobs?

Rating ___ **Comments** _____

Does employee help with others' jobs when needed?

Rating ___ **Comments** _____

Does the employee take direction/criticism well?

Rating ____ **Comments** _____

Additional Comments:

_____

_____

_____

_____

_____

_____

Action Recommended:

_____

_____

_____

_____

_____

_____

Employee Signature: _____ Date: _____

Date of next review: _____

EMPLOYEE SELF-EVALUATION

Instructions:

Rate yourself in each area covered in the self-evaluation using the following scale:

(1) "I need help in this area."
(2) "I am capable, but am currently doing a below average job."
(3) "I am average at this stage."
(4) "I am above average at this."
(5) "I am superior at this."

Rating

1. Self-motivated	1 2 3 4 5
2. Personal appearance	1 2 3 4 5
3. Ability to communicate with clients	1 2 3 4 5
4. Accomplish tasks quickly and accurately	1 2 3 4 5
5. Ability to get along with others	1 2 3 4 5
6. Find ways to minimize loss	1 2 3 4 5
7. Find ways to increase profitability	1 2 3 4 5
8. Alert to animal's condition	1 2 3 4 5
9. Maintain cleanliness and organization (especially in your work area)	1 2 3 4 5
10. Use slack time well	1 2 3 4 5

Signature _____

Date _____ Job Title _____

Individual Employment Contract

Note: The following contract should be used for formatting purposes only. Prior to being signed, the contract should be reviewed by a lawyer in your state to ensure its legality.

INDIVIDUAL EMPLOYMENT CONTRACT

THIS AGREEMENT, signed this ____ day of _____, _____, between _____ , (the "Company"), a veterinary clinic having its principal place of business at _____, _____, _____, _____, and _____, DVM, of _____, _____, _____, _____, (the "EMPLOYEE").

EMPLOYMENT AND BASIC EMPLOYEE DUTIES

1. The Company hereby employs the Employee and the Employee hereby accepts such employment as a staff veterinarian for the term and compensation provided in the following provisions of this Agreement. The Employee agrees that he/she will perform to the Company's satisfaction, such reasonable duties as may from time to time be determined by and assigned to him/her by the executive management of the Company.

2. The Employee represents that he/she has the necessary and adequate competency and ability to perform the duties as may be assigned to him/her by the executive management of the Company. The Employee also expressly agrees as a condition of his/her employment during the term of this Agreement that he/she will devote his/her entire working time, energies and skill to the exclusive service of the Company and to the satisfactory performance of his/her duties in the course of the Company's interests and agrees to accept and perform such other reasonable duties as may be assigned to him/her from time to time by the executive management of the Company.

3. The Company may offer special training in techniques and methods of veterinary medicine and management and the Company may publicize the Employee's association with the Company and if appropriate, the fact that the Employee has such special training or other qualifications.

TERMS OF AGREEMENT

4. Except in the case of earlier termination as specifically provided for in this Agreement, the term of this Agreement shall be effective from _____, _____, through _____, _____, inclusive only.

COMPENSATION

5. For all the services to be rendered by the Employee in any capacity under this Agreement, the Company agrees to pay to the Employee _____ percent (____%) of gross production on all fees charged and collected. Production is only paid on monies actually collected by the company. Production for the sake of this contract will be defined as fees collected for services rendered. The Employee must be involved in the delivery of a given service in order for production compensation to occur. The sale of diet and prescription foods, income generation from boarding, or the sale of pet supplies does not constitute production and therefore, no income is due the Employee from the rendering of these services.

5a. Emergency Service Compensation - In addition to the base salary stated in Paragraph 5, the Employee will also be entitled to additional compensation for after hour emergency service work. After hour emergency service work will be defined, for the purpose of this contract, as cases that have an after hour emergency fee posted on the client statement or work required by the Employee which will require him/her to return to the clinic after regular working hours or work required during weekends and holidays outside of his/her normal work schedule as posted and written by the Company. The Employee will be entitled to the entire after hour emergency fee charged and collected. In addition, the employee will be entitled to _____ percent of those fees charged and collected over and above the after hour emergency fee on services rendered as defined in Section 5 of this Agreement.

5b. The Company further agrees to pay the employee a base salary of no less than _____ dollars ($_____) annually. This guaranteed base is a guarantee of base salary as stated in Clause 5 of this agreement.

6. The Employee hereby acknowledges and agrees that the Company has made no other guarantees or representations with respect to compensation of the Employee.

VACATION TIME

7. The Company agrees to provide a _____ week (___ working days) vacation to the Employee yearly. The Company will not compensate the Employee for said vacation days. Said vacation must be approved by the Company 30 days prior to the requested time. Said vacation must be taken within the contract year or said vacation is forfeited.

PERSONAL HEALTH INSURANCE

8. The Company agrees to obtain and maintain in force a health insurance policy for the Employee during the time the Employee is employed by the Company. The Company will pay the cost of these insurance premiums up to a maximum of _____ dollars per year ($_____). If the cost of the insurance benefit exceeds this maximum amount the Employee will be responsible for the additional premium and this will result as a payroll deduction from the employee's payroll check.

EMERGENCY SERVICE

9. The Employee agrees to participate in the emergency rotation set up by the Company. In the event that any principal of the Company is unable to cover his/her scheduled emergency assignment for reasons of illness, disability, vacation or continuing education seminars, the Employee agrees to fill these vacancies.

PROFESSIONAL LIABILITY/MALPRACTICE INSURANCE

10. The Company agrees to obtain and maintain in force through the AVMA Insurance Plan, a professional liability/malpractice insurance policy for the Employee. Said policy is to be paid for by Company. Policy and limits are to be approved by the Company and will stay in force only as long as the Employee remains employed by the Company under the terms of this agreement.

STATE BUSINESS LICENSE

11. The Company agrees to obtain a state license for the Employee for the state of
_____. The Company agrees to pay the cost for this license during
the term of employment of the Employee. In case of termination, the license fee paid
will be prorated to the last day of employment and an appropriate adjustment will be
made in the Employee's last compensation payment.

HOLIDAYS

12. The Company's operations will be closed to observe the following holidays:

> (a) New Year's Day
>
> (b) Memorial Day
>
> (c) Independence Day
>
> (d) Labor Day
>
> (e) Thanksgiving Day
>
> (f) Christmas Day

The Employee agrees to work _____ (___) of the holidays referred to in
Clause 12, per year. In the event circumstances require other holidays to be worked
by the Employee, the Employee agrees to accept and perform these duties as deemed
necessary by the Company not to exceed _____ (___) such stated holidays during the course of a calendar year.

WORK SCHEDULE

13. The Employee agrees to work an average of _____ hours per week. The
Employee understands that due to the nature of this business, hours will vary from
one week to the next. The Company will strive to schedule the Employee an average
of _____ hours per week and will provide the Employee with ample notice if a substantial change in the work schedule is planned.

CONTINUING EDUCATION

14. The Company agrees to pay for continuing education meetings, up to _____
(___) days, during the course of the calendar year, if approved by the Company prior
to the attendance by the Employee at said meetings. Said payment is for conference
and registration fee only to a maximum of $1,000.00 per contract year.

DUES

15. As an additional benefit to the Employee, the Company agrees to pay for
_____ membership dues.

PERSONAL DAYS

16. The Employee shall be entitled to _____ (___) personal days per contract year. Said personal days will not be compensated to the Employee by the Company.

COVENANT NOT TO COMPETE AND AGREEMENT ON CONFIDENTIALITY

(Not valid in all states.)

17. The Employee agrees that he/she will not own, manage, operate, control, be employed by, participate or be connected in any manner with the ownership, management, operation or control of any business or profession engaged in veterinary services during the term of this Agreement and for a period of _____ (___) years after the termination thereof for any reason, within a _____ (___) mile radius from any of the Company's locations. It is agreed by the Employee that such a reasonable distance shall include, but not be limited to, those towns which are contiguous to the town of _____, _____.

18. The Employee agrees that he/she will not, during the period of this agreement or at any time following the termination of his/her employment with the Company disclose to any person, firm, or corporation the names or addresses of any past, present or prospective clients of the Company or practices of the Company's obtaining business, and will not covertly solicit from any such clients business similar in nature to that performed by the Company. The Employee further agrees not to divulge to any person, firm, or corporation any of the financial affairs of the Company nor to attempt to direct any client away from the Company directly or indirectly.

19. If the Employee violates any of the terms of Clause 17 and/or Clause 18, the Company shall be entitled to an injunction by a competent Court to enjoin and restrain the Employee and each and every other person involved, from continuance of any breach of Clause 17 and/or Clause 18. In addition, the Employee will forfeit any compensation then otherwise due him/her, the said injunction and forfeiture of compensation will be in addition to the Company's right to damages and any other legal remedy which the Company may have due it.

NO FEE VARIANCES

20. The Employee agrees to strictly abide by the current and any future updated fee schedules and policies of the Company as determined from time to time by the executive management of the Company. The lowering or non-application of any minimum fee as set forth in such fee schedules for any services rendered or drugs dispensed will, at the Company's discretion, be deemed conclusively as cause, either for the summary dismissal of the Employee or deduction from the Employee's next compensation payment in an amount equal to the deviation from the minimum fee, or both. The Employee has no authority to adjust a client's statement without the authorization of the Company.

TERMINATION

21. The Employee or the Company may terminate this Agreement at any time upon ninety (90) days' notice in writing to the other. In the event that the Company termi-

nates the employee, the Company shall be obligated in that event to pay the Employee compensation up to the date of termination as long as he/she (the Employee) is still working.

22. If, during the term of this Agreement, the Employee violates the provisions of Clause 1 or 2, the Company may terminate his/her employment on thirty (30) days' notice in writing to the Employee and in that event the Company shall be obligated to pay the Employee his/her compensation up to the date of actual termination.

23. The Company may summarily dismiss the Employee without notice for cause and without limiting the generality thereof, for incompetency, intoxication, insubordination, or cruelty to animals and the Company will endeavor to provide the Employee with written notification of other examples of misconduct which will warrant the Company's acting under this provision.

DEATH OF EMPLOYEE

24. In the event of an Employee's death, this Agreement shall terminate immediately and the Employee's estate shall be paid the Employee's compensation up to the date of death.

SALE OF BUSINESS

25. This Agreement shall terminate in the event that the Company sells its entire operations and the termination shall be effective the date of transfer of the business and the Company shall pay the Employee compensation up to the date of transfer for services rendered by the Employee while he/she was employed under this Agreement.

WAIVER

26. A waiver by either party or breach of any provision of this Agreement shall not operate as or be CONSTRUED as a waiver of any subsequent breach thereof.

NOTICE

27. Any and all notices referred to herein shall be in writing sent by registered mail to the respective parties at the addresses subscribed below following their signatures to this Agreement.

ASSIGNMENT

28. The rights, benefits, and obligations of the Company under this Agreement shall be transferable but the rights, benefits, and obligations of the Employee are entirely personal to the Employee and not transferable by him/her.

ENTIRE AGREEMENT

29. This agreement constitutes the entire agreement between the parties hereto

with respect to the employment of the Employee by the Company and no change in the terms hereof shall be binding unless in writing and duly executed by the parties hereto. Should any part of this Agreement be determined to be void by a competent judicial or legislative authority, the remainder hereto shall remain valid and enforceable.

BENEFIT AND BINDING

30. This Agreement shall be binding upon and inure to the benefit of the Employee and her heirs, executors and administrators and the Company, its successors and assigns.

GOVERNING LAW

31. This Agreement shall be governed by the laws of the State of

_____.

IN WITNESS WHEREOF, the parties have caused this Agreement to be executed in duplicate on the _____ day of _____, _____.

BY: "Employee"   BY: "Company"

_____   _____
(Employee)   *(President/Owner)*

_____   _____
(Signed)   *(Signed)*

_____   _____
Address   Address

_____   _____
City, State, ZIP   City, State, ZIP

Date: _____   Date: _____

WITNESSED:

_____
(Witness)

Date: _____

Practice Name
Address
City, State Zip

HOSPITAL PROCEDURES MANUAL

Effective: _____, _____

This Manual Has Been Prepared For (Name of Employee)

Note: This is only a format manual. A practice's management should review this manual and decide which policies they would like to state for their own practice. Policies, timeframes, and costs can be adjusted.

We want to extend a warm welcome to you as you join our staff at the Practice Name. We hope you'll enjoy working here.

Contained within this manual are policies that pertain to new and present employees alike. It states the hospital's policies on employment, the responsibilities of its employees, and employee benefits.

Again, welcome to our family! If you have any questions or problems, my door is always open to you. If I am not in the hospital and you need to talk to me, please feel free to call me at home.

Practice Manager's Name or Owner Doctor's Name

This Employee Manual is a tool designed to inform you about the relationship you have with (Practice Name) and supersedes in all respects and without exception any prior policies, benefits, or practices of (Practice Name), whether written or not. It is the responsibility of the employee to be familiar with the entire Employee Manual and abide by it.

It may be necessary to amend, supplement, modify or eliminate one or more of the benefits, work rules or policies described in our manual, as well as add new benefits, work rules or policies and we reserve the right to do so, unilaterally, at any time without prior notice.

This manual does not constitute a guarantee of employment for any specified period of time. Employment with (Practice Name) is a voluntary employment-at-will relationship. Nothing in this handbook constitutes an expressed or implied contract of employment or warranty of any benefits. While we hope our working relationship is long and mutually beneficial, you have the right, regardless of any provision or statement appearing in this manual, to terminate your employment relationship with us with or without cause or notice and we reserve the right to do the same.

Incidents of sexual harassment are not condoned and should be reported to the practice manager or hospital owner.

PRACTICE MOTTO
NEVER LET A GOOD CLIENT LEAVE MAD;
SACRIFICE SHORT-TERM DOLLARS FOR LONG TERM PROSPERITY.

MISSION STATEMENT
To provide comprehensive high-quality veterinary care with emphasis on exceptional client service and patient care, while providing employees with desirable, fulfilling and financially rewarding employment.

HOSPITAL PHILOSOPHY
It is our desire to provide the highest quality medical and surgical care to our patients and offer the best possible service to our clients.

Our clients are friends as well as customers, and we value their continued trust and goodwill. Courtesy and patience with clients and their pets are our priorities. An attitude of "We are glad you are here" must be conveyed to each and every client. Clients favor us by selecting us to care for their pets, and not vice versa. This is probably the most important concept for you to remember, and makes it easier to understand the importance of showing genuine concern and interest in a client's problem.

RECRUITMENT AND HIRING

The purpose of staff recruitment activities is to attract the best-qualified and competent candidates for employment with the hospital. Applications are evaluated according to the requirements of the job and the knowledge, skills, abilities and personal characteristics possessed.

INTRODUCTORY PERIOD

The first three months of employment will be an introductory period for all employees. During this time, an employee is ineligible for any hospital benefits. At the end of the introductory period, performance will be reviewed and if it is deemed satisfactory, the employee will be placed on regular status. At this time, the employee will be eligible for benefits which apply to his or her employment status. If it is apparent that performance is not satisfactory and training or counseling has not resulted in sufficient progress during the introductory period, an employee may be terminated without advance notice.

EMPLOYMENT POLICIES

It is the policy of this hospital to treat all applicants and employees equally without regard to race, religion, age, color, ancestry, sex, national origin, veteran status, or handicap.

DISCRIMINATION COMPLAINT

Our hospital has a Discrimination Complaint System through which an employee may report any situation that he or she feels is discriminatory. As with other job-related problems, the problem should first be discussed with a supervisor. However, the complaint may be taken directly to the Practice Manager. If after initial discussion the problem is not resolved satisfactorily, a Discrimination Complaint Form may be filed. A copy of this form will be forwarded to the Practice Manager who will determine what action is to be taken.

HARASSMENT

Our practice is committed to providing a work environment that is free of discrimination. This policy prohibits harassment in any form, including verbal, physical and sexual harassment.

Any employee who believes he or she has been harassed by a co-worker, manager or agent of the employer is to immediately report any such incident to the employer. The employer will investigate and take appropriate action.

NON-SOLICITATION POLICY (Optional)

It is the policy of this hospital to prohibit internal solicitation among employees, as well as outside solicitors. This policy has been established to help protect the working environment and to avoid uncomfortable situations that may develop.

EMERGENCY PROCEDURES

In Case of Fire

Employees on duty are to call _____ and inform the emergency service of the situation. Be sure to tell them the hospital name, address and location of fire. If the fire is not life threatening, one individual should try to extinguish or contain the fire with the appropriate fire extinguishers, while other employees move patients to a safe area in the hospital.

If there appears to be no safe area in the hospital, patients should be moved outside to employees' cars, tied to fences, or placed in _____. The practice manager and owner should be contacted as soon as possible.

In Case of Accident
The injury should be treated by the employee's physician as soon as possible. Also, any on-the-job injury should be reported to the Practice Manager as soon as possible.

EMPLOYMENT STATUS

Various statuses of employment have been defined as follows:
Introductory Period: The first three months of an individual's employment.
Full-time Employee: An employee who works an average of 35 hours or more over a period of six consecutive months.
Part-time Employee: An employee who works less than an average of 35 hours per week over a period of six consecutive months.

HOSPITAL STAFF POLICIES

Promptness in reporting to work is a basic requirement.
The personal use of the telephone during working hours is discouraged. All incoming and outgoing personal calls are to be kept to a bare minimum. You can return calls on your time (during lunch or after you are clocked out). No personal long distance phone calls are to be made except in case of emergency situations.
Personal pets are to be brought into the clinic only if they are ill, need medical attention, or under extenuating circumstances. They are to be treated during the employee's off time.
Unemployed personnel, (i.e. friends, family, etc., of hospital staff members) are not to be present within the hospital at any time without prior approval of the Practice Manager.
There will be no moonlighting, (i.e., work undertaken outside the hospital) in any occupation pertaining to animal care or services without written approval of the Practice Manager.
No smoking is allowed in the hospital at any time. The chewing of gum is restricted from the public areas of the hospital.

PAY DAYS

Employees are paid bi-weekly. Payroll checks will be available no later than 4:00 p.m. every other Friday.

TIME CARDS

All employees are required to keep a time card record of their work, observing the following practices:
Record your time in and time out as you initiate and conclude your work duties daily.
Record time accurately.
Record any breaks in the workday (i.e., lunch, medical appointments, personal time that was taken off) and make a note of it on the time card.
Any swapping of hours with another employee or substituting of days off must be approved two weeks in advance prior to this arrangement by the Practice Manager.
We try to see that everyone receives a minimum of one hour for lunch; however, if business is pushed and the hospital is behind in its work, a shortened lunch period will be required. If the schedule permits, longer lunch times are permitted.
Part-time or full-time personnel who are hired to work weekends and holidays will be expected to work each weekend or holiday as assigned, including weekends of holidays or special events.
Employees are required to sign their time cards at the conclusion of each pay

week before payroll checks are issued.

OVERTIME
All overtime work must be authorized in advance by the Practice Manager. You will be paid time and one-half for authorized hours worked in excess of forty hours in one week.

WORK SCHEDULES
Work schedules are posted two weeks in advance. Once the schedule has been posted for 24 hours, it will be considered final. Changes in the assigned work schedule other than vacations or personal leave can only be made with three weeks prior permission of the Practice Manager. Employees requesting a change of schedule are responsible for arranging for a substitute of equivalent skill and experience from within the existing hospital staff and must receive both verbal approval and written approval on the work schedule for said substitution from the Practice Manager.

In emergency or dire stress situations, it may be necessary to occasionally change the planned staff work schedule, possibly with only a last minute's notice given, in order to meet the hospital's case load and to provide service to our patients and clients. It is expected that all hospital staff members will be aware of this possible inconvenience to their personal schedules and will conduct themselves in a cooperative, professional manner.

ATTENDANCE
Punctuality and regular attendance are essential to the proper operation of any business. They also help you establish a good working reputation. All employees are expected to report promptly for the work time scheduled and should plan on arriving at least five (5) minutes before the stated time for work to begin in order to be prepared for work at the appropriate time. An employee not ready to work at his/her required/expected time constitutes tardiness. All employees are expected to be prompt and punctual.

Any tardy employee should have his/her time card initialed by the veterinarian in charge. An explanation should be noted on the time card.

If you are unable to work for any reason, please notify the Practice Manager by telephone or in person as early as possible before starting time. DO NOT call and leave a message on the recorder.

PERSONNEL RECORDS
It is your responsibility to insure that your personnel records are kept up-to-date. This includes notification of changes in address, name, marital status, number of dependents, telephone number, or anything else you feel the hospital should know.

Your personnel file is a consolidation of information throughout your employment with the hospital. It is treated in a highly confidential manner and only authorized people are permitted to review it. You may see your file upon request.

CLIENT RELATIONS/HOSPITAL RECORDS
Any breach in the confidentiality of client information will not be tolerated. All client records, including charts, radiographs, financial information, etc., are confidential and are the legal property of the hospital.

Medical records are legal documents. All appropriate information including medical, financial and brief documentation of pertinent client conversations must be documented legally to provide a comprehensive record. Deletions or changes to a record may be done with only one line through the word or sentence to be changed.

MEDIA

Employees are to make no statements, nor provide any information to be used by newspapers, television or radio stations or any other media. Reporters requesting information should be referred to the doctor in charge or the practice manager.

TREATMENT OF PATIENTS

Our hospital policy is that we treat a client's pet as if it were our own. Humane treatment of animals is absolutely demanded of each employee. Any type of animal abuse will be the basis for immediate termination without notice.

EMPLOYEE BENEFITS

Vacation

Full-time employees will receive a one-week (5 day) vacation at the completion of their first and second year of employment at (Practice Name). A two-week (10 day) vacation may be taken by full-time employees at the completion of their third year of employment and all subsequent years of employment thereafter up to seven years.

Any employee who is employed by the hospital for more than seven years will be entitled to a three-week (15 day) vacation. Vacation days are not cumulative. That is, vacation days may not be saved from one year to use in the next. Any vacation days not used during the calendar year (January to December) will be lost and will not be compensated. Vacations must be scheduled and approved at least one month prior to vacation period.

Vacation days taken immediately prior to, during, or after a holiday must be approved two weeks in advance by the Practice Manager.

Sick Time

Full-time employees will accumulate sick time at the rate of 1/2 day per month from the date of employment, but these days may not be used until the employee has worked for the practice for at least three months. Sick days will be cumulative. That is, sick days not used within one calendar year will carry over into the next year to a maximum of twelve (12) days. After 12 sick days have been accumulated, employees will be paid for sick days not used, in excess of 12 days, during the last week in December. However, sick days may not be used to extend vacation time. Sick time is just that and is not to be abused in any fashion. Sick time is provided for the benefit of our employees. If an employee becomes ill, he or she may need the extra time. Any employee found abusing sick time will be dealt with on an individual basis.

Personal Leave (Option To Sick Leave)

Full-time employees will accumulate personal leave, which may be used for sick leave, at the rate of one-half (1/2) day per month or a total of six days per year from the date of employment, upon successful completion of the introductory period, but these days may not be used until the employee has worked full-time for (Practice Name) for at least three months. Prorated personal leave (as previously described) may be cumulative for two years, for a maximum of 12 days, and if not used within this 24 month calendar period, you will be paid for those days or hours that were not used. This will be like a bonus at the end of the year for good health. Accrued personal leave days may be used to extend vacation days if the above requirements have been met.

Holidays

For our purposes, there will be seven paid holidays during the year. They are New Year's Day, Memorial Day, July 4th, Labor Day, Thanksgiving Day and Christmas (or the Jewish New Year), as well as each employee's own birthday. The birthday holiday is an extra benefit and will be paid only if the day is not worked. We cannot pay double time for this holiday if it is worked by an employee. Full-time employees are entitled to one day's pay for each holiday. If an employee is scheduled to work on a holiday, he or she will receive double time for that day (regular pay for hours worked plus holiday pay for these hours). The Practice Manager must be notified at least two weeks in advance of posting the schedule when an employee plans to take a day off for his or her birthday.

Part-time employees are not entitled to holiday benefits; however, if a part-time employee works on a holiday, he or she will receive double time for those hours worked.

If a holiday falls on a day that the employee is not normally scheduled to work, the employee will not receive any additional compensation for that day. The holiday benefit is paid only if the employee would normally have been paid for the day, but since the hospital was closed, they were unable to work.

Staff Entertainment and Education Functions

As deemed possible and financially affordable, the hospital will provide special social/entertainment or educational functions for the staff either in a partial or total capacity when possible.

Health Insurance

Medical Insurance is available through _____ Insurance Company. Premiums vary depending on an individual's sex and age. Your total monthly premium is estimated to be $_____ . This premium may be paid in part by the hospital.

At the time of the initial three-month review and at the yearly reviews that take place thereafter and at the discretion of the hospital, an option will be given to the employee to subsidize insurance premiums or receive monetary raises. Additional subsidization can be made in lieu of raises or along with them as employment continues.

Part-time employees may purchase insurance through the hospital but they will be responsible for the full premium. Coverage is available for $_____ per month for a single person.

Spouse and dependent coverage is also available through the hospital; however, employees will be responsible for the premium differential if such coverage is desired.

Life Insurance

As part of _____ Insurance Company's policy, the employee will also receive a life insurance policy. This is normally a $10,000 term life insurance policy. At the time an employee becomes eligible for this benefit, an informational brochure will be provided explaining this policy and the benefits available.

Veterinary Services At Reduced Rate (Option 1)

After the three-month introductory period, all employees, both full and part-time, will be entitled to a 50% discount on all medical and surgical services with the exception of those listed below. This benefit applies only to those animals personally owned by the employee. This benefit is limited to three pets per employee. In order to receive this benefit, all services are to be paid for when rendered.

Boarding	20% Off Standard Fees
Baths and Dips	20% Off Standard Fees
Grooming	Full Price
Prescription Diets	10% Over Cost

Veterinary Services At Reduced Rate (Option 2)

Full-time employees will receive care for their animal(s) at no charge up to a maximum indicated in the following schedule:

After 3 months of employment	$100
After 1 year of employment	$200
After 2 years of employment	$300
After 3 years of employment	$400
After 5 years of employment	$500

This figure is based on the hospital's current charges for any procedures performed by the doctor. After this maximum is met, a 50% discount will be given on all additional service.

Staff Veterinary Medical Care Benefits (Option 3)

After the three-month introductory period, all employees, both full-time and part-time, will be entitled to a discount on almost all hospital and veterinary services. All hospital professional services and supplies will be discounted to essentially hospital cost (50% for full-time employees and 25% for part-time employees) with the exception of the following:

Boarding	20% Off Standard Fees
Baths And Dips	20% Off Standard Fees
Grooming	Full Price
Prescription Diets	10% Over Cost

Please keep in mind that this discount policy applies only to your personally owned pets. In order to qualify for the discount, you must make sure specific records are pulled by the receptionists and that thorough notations are made on the record by the attending veterinarian. Your personally owned pets must be listed or registered with the hospital both upon initially gaining employment and at the end of the three-month introductory period in order to qualify for the employee discount.

Secondly, as a bonus for longevity, full-time employees will receive medical care for their animals at no charge up to the maximum indicated in the following schedule:

After 1 year of employment	$100
After 2 years of employment	$200
After 3 years of employment	$300
After 5 years of employment	$500

After the above amounts have been used, the standard 50% discount applies. This figure is based on the hospital's current charges for any procedures performed by the doctor. After this maximum is met, a 50% discount will be given on all additional services. All services are to be paid for when rendered. Upon termination of employment, leave of absence or vacation, payment of any balance is expected before receiving the final paycheck. Employees are expected to assist in procedures on their animals on their own time. All procedures should be performed before or after the employee's scheduled shift or on his/her day off. If any procedures are performed during the employee's regular working hours, employees must punch out for that time. Regular part-time employees will also receive these benefits, their maximum being 50% of those above (i.e. a 25% discount).

The latter benefits are specific only to the veterinary medical care benefits and may not be considered transferable to other employee benefit areas. In addition, the medical/surgical treatments of the staff's personally owned pets are to adhere to the hospital's routine protocol for these services and are to be provided under the direction of the on-duty doctor.

Thirdly, an employee who is performing well at the time of his annual performance review may also elect to receive a portion of his salary increase in the form of increased veterinary benefits. Additional veterinary benefits can be made in lieu of raises or along with them as employment continues.

Uniform Reimbursement

Hospital employees will wear the proper uniform for their respective positions. Full-time employees will be reimbursed the cost of a uniform to a maximum of $100 per year, and part-time employees will be reimbursed to a maximum of $50 per year.

Smocks are provided for the protection of both part-time and full-time employees' clothing, as well as maintaining a professional appearance. A name tag is also provided for all staff members.

UNIFORMS AND GROOMING

The professional atmosphere of the hospital is to be maintained by all employees while present in the hospital. Employees are expected to be dressed according to the hospital uniform code, to be well groomed and to maintain their uniforms in a clean state at all times.

Hospital employees will wear the proper uniform for their respective positions:

Female Technicians: White pants, choice of shirt or blouse, white shoes, and a hospital approved jacket.

Male Technicians: White pants, choice of shirt, white shoes, and a hospital-approved jacket.

Receptionist: A hospital approved color professional jacket, white pants, choice of shirt or blouse, and white shoes.

Female Animal Handlers: A hospital approved color professional jacket, choice of blouse, navy blue pants, and blue or white shoes.

Male Animal Handlers: Navy blue pants, a hospital approved color professional jacket, choice of shirt, and blue or white shoes.

SURGICAL GREENS ARE NOT TO BE WORN BY THE STAFF.

EMPLOYEE REVIEWS

Each employee will be reviewed at the end of his or her introductory period and a salary adjustment, if deemed appropriate, will be made at that time. Reviews will be made thereafter on a yearly basis with appropriate salary adjustments.

Raises will be given based on an employee's performance, work attitude, attendance record, responsiveness and willingness to work. A sample of the employee performance evaluation form used will be provided to each employee.

EMPLOYEE INCENTIVE PROGRAM

An employee incentive program was implemented to further help the hospital market services to its clients and ensure that our patients are kept up-to-date on routine preventative procedures.

The basis of compensation will be 10 percent of the increase in gross income, or X. Each employee is evaluated based on their performance. For this, a specific employee evaluation form will be used. An employee can score 0 to 100 on this evaluation. The score will then be the basis for the distribution of bonus money. If an employee is working 35 hours or more per week, which is considered full time, they would then receive their appropriate share of the bonus fund. If an employee is working less than 35 hours per week and is considered part-time, the bonus must be proportionately reduced, which is another calculation that would be done once their evaluation score was determined. The evaluations will occur quarterly.

An example of this formula and calculation would be as follows:

Employee	Evaluation Score
April	40
Judy	70
Jack	80
Claire	100
Total Of Scores	290

X or the total bonus money (10% of the increased gross) is then divided by the total score. The resulting figure is then multiplied by the employee's score to get the dollar bonus figure.

If, for example, X equaled $500, then $500 / 290 = 1.72 and the following table would apply:

Employee	1.72 x Evaluation Score =	Bonus Amount
April	1.72 x 40 =	$68.80
Judy	1.72 x 70 =	$120.40
Jack	1.72 x 80 =	$137.60
Claire	1.72 x 80 =	$172.00

Total Employee Bonus $498.80

The figure of 1.72 is then used until the next evaluation, at which time a new figure will be calculated. This incentive program is based on productivity and an individual employee's performance. If the hospital does not realize a profit in a given quarter, or if an employee does not receive a favorable evaluation, a bonus will not be paid.

An employee must be employed during the entire quarter in order to be eligible for a bonus. If an employee is hired during the quarter or leaves their employment for any reason during the quarter, they are not entitled to any bonus funds. This is an all or nothing program.

LEAVE OF ABSENCE
A leave of absence may be requested for maternity, extended illness or extenuating circumstances. Requests will be considered on an individual basis. If an employee is granted a leave of absence, he or she will be reinstated upon return to the same position that was held prior to their leave of absence.

HAZARDOUS MATERIALS
This hospital feels responsible for providing its staff with a safe and healthful workplace. The providing of safety equipment and information is the primary means of accomplishing this commitment. The hospital tries to monitor all functional areas to make sure there are no hazards and that compliance with all federal, state and local health and safety codes is maintained.

During the performance of your job, you may come in contact with chemicals or other hazardous materials. Each of these materials has its own properties and characteristics. Chemicals in any form can be stored, handled, and used safely, if their properties and characteristics are understood and proper safeguards are taken.

This hospital has, in compliance with OSHA's Employee Right To Know law, all of the Material Safety Data Sheets (MSDS's) for the materials that are used on the premises, as well as a list of the materials on hand and a hazardous material handling plan. These documents contain information which describes the normal day-to-day handling of chemicals, as well as what to do for accidental spills or emergencies.

The hazardous material handling plan, inventory list, and MSDS's are located _____. If you wish to examine any of these documents, please feel free to ask your supervisor for time to do so.

We need your help in keeping up to date. If, during your daily duties, you notice any chemical that is not on the inventory list maintained in the front of the MSDS book, please notify your supervisor immediately so that it may be evaluated and proper safety precautions implemented.

HONESTY

The hospital expects all employees to be as fair to it as it is to them. The removal of any hospital property from the premises is not acceptable behavior. It is expected that all employees will be aware of this and will monitor themselves as well as others. It is also expected that the privacy and integrity of clients, doctors and other staff will be respected. Any conversation, discussions or other information gathered from the hospital is to remain in the hospital.

Gossip and disparaging remarks regarding clients or fellow staff members will not be tolerated and can subject an employee to suspension or termination.

DISCIPLINE

All discipline shall be dispensed in the following manner:

The first altercation shall be addressed by verbal warning.

The second altercation shall be addressed by a written and witnessed reprimand.

Any further altercations will lead to suspension without pay, or immediate dismissal, if all of the above have taken place in any three-month period.

Discipline pertains to any and all company policy.

TERMINATION

An employee who voluntarily leaves his or her employment at (Practice Name) is required to provide a two-week notice and work his or her hours during this time period. Those employees who are terminated for cause or willful misconduct (see below) will be discharged immediately and without further compensation. Individuals terminated for other reasons will be discharged immediately, but two weeks' severance pay and compensation for vacation time will be given.

Misconduct includes such things as: excessive tardiness, excessive absenteeism, careless conduct or negligence, leaving the hospital without approval, dishonesty, insubordination, consumption of or being under the influence of drugs or alcohol, theft, unapproved use of company premises or property, possession or use of weapons, defacement of company property, physical assault on another employee or visitor, battery, divulging confidential information, violation of company rules, or previously stated unacceptable conduct.

SUMMARY OF HOSPITAL AND STAFF POLICIES

Your employment at (Practice Name) is based on a mutual agreement, the fulfillment of which rests upon good faith, acceptance and performance of job responsibilities, and fair and reasonable business conduct.

The hospital and its staff members are here to provide a service to our clients and to make our clients feel at home. Always keep in mind that the clients who come to our hospital with their pets are the reason that we exist. Therefore, never underestimate the power of one client in relation to this total business.

It is extremely important to attempt to maintain a good relationship with both your fellow staff members and clients. Personalities of people will be different, and we must learn to respect the viewpoint of others.

OPEN DOOR POLICY

The policies and procedures set down in this manual have been stated to help you better understand your duties and responsibilities as well as the benefits of employment at our hospital. I greatly appreciate my staff and their commitment to this hospital and the patients' welfare. In an effort to maintain our high quality of patient care and optimum work environment, your input and involvement are necessary and requested.

My door is always open to you. Feel free to contact me at any time. Together we can achieve the goals we all desire.

_____

Practice Manager

_____

Owner-Doctor

_____

Employee Signature

_____

Date

Employee signature is to acknowledge receipt of handbook and further to acknowledge that this is not a contract, but instead, a statement of policies and procedures and is in no way to be interpreted as a contract of employment.

Notes

Notes

Notes